P9-CKP-365

Death ar

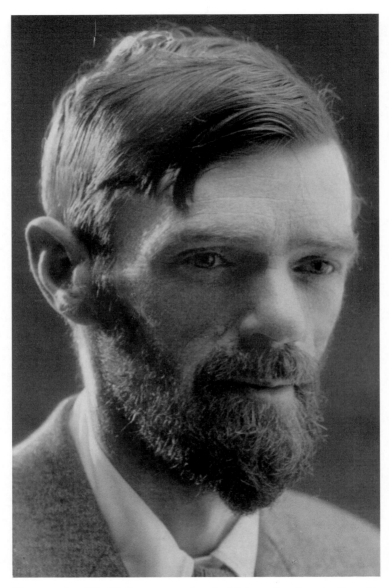

Photograph of D. H. Lawrence taken in Majorca by Ernesto Guardia in 1929

Death and the Author

Author

How D. H. Lawrence Died,
and was Remembered

David Ellis

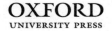

OXFORD
UNIVERSITY PRESS

OXFORD
UNIVERSITY PRESS

Great Clarendon Street, Oxford ox2 6dp

Oxford University Press is a department of the University of Oxford.
It furthers the University's objective of excellence in research, scholarship,
and education by publishing worldwide in

Oxford New York

Auckland Cape Town Dar es Salaam Hong Kong Karachi
Kuala Lumpur Madrid Melbourne Mexico City Nairobi
New Delhi Shanghai Taipei Toronto

With offices in

Argentina Austria Brazil Chile Czech Republic France Greece
Guatemala Hungary Italy Japan Poland Portugal Singapore
South Korea Switzerland Thailand Turkey Ukraine Vietnam

Oxford is a registered trade mark of Oxford University Press
in the UK and in certain other countries

Published in the United States
by Oxford University Press Inc., New York

British Library Cataloguing in Publication Data

Data available

Library of Congress Cataloging in Publication Data

Data available

Typeset by SPI Publisher Services, Pondicherry, India
Printed in Great Britain
on acid-free paper by
Clays Ltd, St Ives plc

ISBN 978-0-19-954665-7

1 3 5 7 9 10 8 6 4 2

In memoriam: D. J. Enright

Contents

Part III. Remembrance

Introduction

S hakespeare has some shrewd comments on the way many of us cope with death. In the second part of his *Henry IV*, Justice Shallow is excitedly waiting with his cousin Silence for the arrival of Falstaff and thinking of all the acquaintances of his youth who are now no more. When Silence tells him 'We shall all follow, cousin', he replies, 'Certain, 'tis certain; very sure, very sure. Death, as the psalmist sayeth, is certain to all; all shall die. How a good yoke of bullocks at Stamford Fair?' Shallow is an old man and exhibits an immediately recognizable characteristic of human nature in wanting to distract himself from the thought of his own approaching dissolution with everyday affairs. This is much easier now than it was for the Elizabethans, threatened with periodic outbursts of plague and familiar as they were, in an age of far lower life-expectancy, with the untimely deaths of children, relatives, and friends. In their quasi-compulsory church-going they would also be accustomed to hearing various texts directing attention to death's inevitability, including the one from Psalm 89 which Shallow echoes: 'What man is he that liveth, and shall not see death?' The Church provided comfort against the terrors of dying although it also strengthened its power by adding to those terrors a fear of the Last Judgement.

In our time, when there is news of anti-ageing pills which will make four score and ten seem like middle age, and the processes of dying have been largely hidden from us, it is not so difficult to keep the mind focused on the price of bullocks at Stamford Fair. And yet, because what the Psalmist says still holds good, there may be occasions when we would rather be reconciled to its truth than distracted from it. Now that for many of us the Church can no longer provide that function, one possibly important resource is biography: the record of the experience of our fellow mortal creatures.

In one of his lives of the poets, Dr Johnson describes Addison's lack of success in trying to reform a young relative of 'very irregular life, and perhaps of loose opinions'. When he found his life drawing to a close, Addison called for the young man and apparently said: 'I have sent for you that you may see how a Christian may die.' In the nineteenth century the religious journals were full of accounts of people who had died the good, Christian death in the Addisonian fashion. These conjure up a world which is largely alien to us, although there were glimpses of it at the time of the last Pope's death. Reporting in a radio broadcast on the heroic struggles of John Paul II with a large number of life-threatening conditions, and his refusal to contemplate surrender, one Vatican watcher related those struggles to a debate in the United States over mercy-killing and the opposition there had been to doctors who wanted to disconnect the life-support machines of a terminally ill patient. It was the Pope's aim, the observer suggested, to leave Roman Catholics with one final lesson in the manner of his dying.

One does not have to be either a Catholic or a Christian to believe that accounts of death may still serve some useful, exemplary function and help reconcile us to the certainty of our own: that this is part of what Johnson once called, in a famous *Rambler* essay, the uses and dignity of biography. But for this to be possible the accounts need to be reasonably accurate and not distorted in order to conform to some predetermined pattern. A scholar investigating those good Christian deaths of the nineteenth century has found that there are sometimes significant discrepancies between what was said in public and what can be discovered from letters, journals, and memoirs. It might be argued that this is not important if the records served their purpose and that in these matters fiction serves just as well as truth. No one wanting to reflect on death could feel short-changed by what Tolstoy has to say on the matter in his powerful and disturbing novella *The Death of Ivan Ilyich*. Yet that work never pretends to be anything other than a story, so that any reservations one might have—that there may be moments in the narrative, for example, when the author appears to have gone too far out of his way to darken the picture—are complaints which relate to what one might call its truth to life and not of course its truth to the lived experience of any particular individual Tolstoy happened to know. *The Death of Ivan Ilyich* is quite clearly not fiction masquerading as biography, a genre of limited usefulness (as well as dignity), especially after the masquerade has been exposed. It does make a difference to discover that not all those celebrated in the religious journals did in fact die in mild resignation to the will of God and with cheering, edificatory words for those around them. Truth in biography may often prove an impossible ideal but when biographers cease to live by it, forgetting or ignoring what can be known in order to achieve a moral purpose, that purpose is devalued.

Accurate, detailed reports of what people feel as they are dying, and what close observers make of their deaths, are hard to come by. There is an obvious advantage therefore in focusing on the lives (and deaths) of writers, since they tend not only to be much written about, but also expert in describing their own attitudes and feelings. Yet for there to be the kind of abundance of information which fills out the picture and allows for cross-checking, the writers have to be relatively recent. This is only one of several reasons why the focus in this experiment in biography is on D. H. Lawrence, who died when he was only 44 and for whom death was always an important topic. Many other writers are discussed but it is around his experience, and the response of others to it, that the material is chiefly organized.

Some philosophers maintain that, as we can never ourselves know what death is, nothing can be said about it, and they also argue that expressions like 'I'd rather be dead' make no sense since they involve a comparison one of whose terms is something of which we are necessarily ignorant. ('Whenever we make the attempt to imagine our death', writes Freud, we can on reflection perceive that 'we really survive as spectators'.) All this may be true but only if the word death is taken to mean being dead: non-existent, whereas in its ordinary use the word tends to include dying and on that topic we are all likely to become experienced, although some more than others. At the age of 59 the French novelist Stendhal collapsed in a Paris street and never recovered consciousness. Lawrence, on the other hand, was dogged by both pulmonary tuberculosis and chronic bronchitis during the last five or six years of his life and had plenty of time to see death coming: his illnesses gave him the opportunity to develop feelings and attitudes about dying which Stendhal did not need and may not have had.

How people respond to the news that they have an illness for which there is likely to be no cure is one of the implicit themes of this book. So also is the attitude they might adopt to medicine, orthodox or unorthodox, and the difference between the retention of a positive attitude to an illness and what is now called denial. Other themes are the stereotyping that accompanies serious illness—throughout the nineteenth century and beyond, a long list of quite specific attributes would be conjured up by the word 'consumptive'—and the anger the sick feel when they believe that their death will represent the triumph of their enemies. There is also that anger at having to leave the world too soon, which is represented so vividly by Tolstoy's Ivan Ilyich. Because the attitude of individuals to dying will obviously be influenced by their religious convictions and whether or not they believe in an after-life, that has had to be one of the concerns. The moment of death is of obvious significance and so too is that institution which goes with it of famous last words. After those words, the subject's own testimony is clearly no longer available since what follows death is an undiscovered country from whose bourn no traveller returns, as Hamlet famously said (rather forgetting his father). But there are other relevant witnesses to the difficulties of burial, the nature of bereavement, the complications which often arise over a will, and to the problem of how best to remember someone who has been much loved or admired. Most people now feel that the only chance they have of living on after death is in the minds of those who survive them but, in the case of famous writers, there is often a bitter struggle over image rights: a conflict between survivors as to how the dead should be remembered. Words are then sometimes uttered or written which would make the objects of dispute turn in their graves if the assumption of their ability to do so did not demonstrate once again how natural and yet false it is to imagine death, not as the physical extinction it really is, but a state of animation temporarily suspended.

These are some of the aspects of death, dying, and remembrance treated in this book. Although they are important, they are not biographical topics as obviously appealing as others: the sex life of the subject, for example; but then what is biography *for* if it does not try to explore all of the issues which might matter to us? In doing that, and with a detailed particularity not always possible in the more usual cradle-to-grave biography, there is a risk of seeming morbidly or unpleasantly intrusive. In *Lady Chatterley's Lover*, the heroine finds herself fascinated by the gossip of the nurse, Mrs Bolton, but afterwards feels a little ashamed: 'She ought not to listen with this queer rabid curiosity. After all, one may hear the most private affairs of other people, but only in a spirit of respect for the struggling, battered thing which any human soul is.' Gossip is different from biography, even if it is sometimes hard to detect where the difference lies; but in both, natural human curiosity needs to be accompanied by the respect Lawrence talks about here.

It is never easy to strike the right note, to be neither too flippant nor too solemn where either the death of an individual or death in general is concerned. Two of D. J. Enright's more distinguished contemporaries simultaneously illustrated and overcame the problem when in 1983 they both reviewed the *Oxford Book of Death* which he had edited. John Carey wrote a witty account, borrowing from the Enright anthology Woody Allen's well-known remark that he was not afraid to die but did not want to be there when it happened. He noted how statistics of mortality would suggest that a few of the people who began to read his review would have passed away by the middle of it, but for those who remained Carey quoted Leopardi's conviction that death is not really painful because in the final stages 'Nature dulls the areas of sensation'. 'Personally', he then continued, 'I'd prefer assurance on that point from someone with firsthand experience, though I quite see it's difficult to arrange.' In contrast to Carey, Phillip Larkin largely eschewed the gallows humour which death so often excites and concentrated instead on the remarkable talent human beings have for ignoring, or (like Shallow) distracting themselves from, the certainty of their future extinction. This he regarded as such a necessary condition of living that a book about death seemed to him a foolhardy enterprise. He concluded that 'in the last analysis the intrusion of death into our lives is so ruthless, so irreversible, so rarely unaccompanied by pain, terror and remorse, that to "anthologise" it . . . seems at best irrelevant, at worst an error of taste' and he reminded his readers of La Rochefoucauld's conviction that 'Death and the sun are not to be looked at steadily'.

It may well be that death is a phenomenon which it is impossible to meet face to face, that we always have to take furtive glimpses at it through our fingers, as when trying to look at a bright sun. But the aim in this book is not a direct contact with death and dying but to make those topics more familiar through proxy (the third topic of remembrance is a different matter since it is one where, as Larkin puts it in his review, the pressure eases). This tactic may of course have been regarded by Larkin as no less an error of taste than the *Oxford Book of Death*. The Victorians had a concern with all the circumstances of our dying, which can now seem morbid and obsessive. We by contrast are accustomed to ignoring death or taking it in our stride, except when it happens to be our own. Although this may suggest that we have more taste than they had, it may also indicate that the pendulum has now swung too far the other way. After all, only dyed-in-the-wool solipsists can believe that objects which they cannot bear to look at, or have too much taste to notice, must therefore have ceased to exist.

Part I
Dying

Bandol

Most mornings he would spend propped up in bed, nursing his decreasing strength or battling with one of his frequent chills. From his bedroom he could look directly out on to the Mediterranean where he liked to imagine the Argonauts, or Odysseus calling the commands as he steered past the 'foamy islands' just beyond the bay. What he could actually see was the occasional ocean liner heading east toward Cannes, 'like a small beetle walking the edge', and leaving behind 'a long thread of dark smoke | like a bad smell'.

When he felt fit enough he would struggle down to the edge of the water only fifty yards away. His illnesses had so reduced his lung capacity and his strength that longer walks were increasingly out of the question. In his younger days he had been, like many of his contemporaries, a prodigious walker, thinking nothing of fifteen or twenty miles on a Sunday outing. On three occasions he had crossed the Alps largely on foot, averaging during one of these expeditions twenty-five miles uphill on consecutive days. But now the briefest excursion tired him out. Another obvious symptom was a persistent cough, with a good deal of accompanying phlegm. To the dismay of visitors, he would carry with him a batch of used envelopes which he discreetly spat into and then returned to his pocket with the relative indifference of a man who blows his nose because he has a cold. His manner with all but those very close to him was to behave as if nothing was seriously wrong. At no point did he try to elicit sympathy by presenting himself to the outside world as an invalid. His father, a powerful man habituated to feeling healthy, had been easily alarmed when he became ill and prone to a self-pity which his stern mother had schooled her son to despise.

Even in winter there were flowers everywhere you looked in Bandol. Up until Christmas 1929, he was able to enjoy late-flowering yellow narcissi which were grown commercially in the field next to his house. Flowers had always been one of his passions, a strong initial interest bolstered by academic study. At school, and then later when he was training to be a teacher, botany had been one of his best subjects. It was the profusion and variety of the wild flowers in the area around the small seaside resort which had helped to confirm his liking for it when he had first arrived there in November 1928, almost a year before. He and his wife had then stayed in a hotel, the Beau Rivage, and been happy there. He had enjoyed wandering down to the port to watch the fishing boats come in, 'silvery loads of sardines glittering on the sands of the shores'; and he liked observing the life in the town even when, as he at one point sardonically noted, it chiefly consisted of dogs.

It was because he had then been so contented but also so relatively well in Bandol that he had come back there in September 1929. He had developed a superstitious attachment to those places where he had experienced relief from his condition and a corresponding distaste for those which had been the scene of some crisis. For a year in the mid-1920s he had lived in the top half of a beautiful old house outside Florence, the Villa Mirenda, with spectacular views over the Tuscan hills. But after he suffered a massive haemorrhage there, it lost much of its charm for him. One might have thought that the Beau Rivage would also have lost its charm when shortly after his first arrival he discovered that his former friend Katherine Mansfield had also stayed there, before she was diagnosed with tuberculosis and later in an early phase of her unsuccessful struggle against it. But then, as he frequently insisted to his many correspondents, it was not tuberculosis which was seriously troubling him but a more mundane condition: not his lungs but his 'miserable bronchials'. He was not so much suffering, that is, from the disease which every year was proving fatal to tens of thousands of his contemporaries, many of them still young or, like him, in early middle age, but rather from one of the ill-defined chest complaints endemic in the small Midlands mining town in which he had grown up. As he knew from experience, these could often be chronic without proving fatal.

When he came back to Bandol he would have willingly continued to stay at the Beau Rivage but his wife was sick of hotel life and felt they needed a house. She hankered after what he had called, during a phase of their wanderings which had taken them to Australia, a little 'ome of her own. The house they chose was named Beau Soleil. It was a considerable come-down from the Mirenda, or from the Fontana Vecchia, the villa they had rented in Taormina when they had lived in Sicily for more than two years at the beginning of the 1920s. It was also very different from their ranch house in New Mexico which was certainly poky and primitive (no electricity, no running water), but which stood high in the mountains above Taos, looking down on the Rio Grande.

He had named it Kiowa after an Indian tribe which had once camped in the area and it gave not the slightest hint of suburbia. The Beau Soleil, on the other hand, had had about as much attention devoted to its architecture as its name, and was an early sign of that development which would turn all the once-charming towns or villages on the French Riviera into housing estates for those with money to burn. On first seeing it, their old friend Norman Douglas called it 'one of those dreadful little bungalows of gaudy cardboard', but there may be times in life when what it feels like to live in a house is more important than what it looks like from outside. The interior decorations were not in fact much to his taste, suggestive in their vulgar elaboration (he and his wife thought) of what a rich man might provide for his mistress, for a *femme entretenue*. But in addition to the advantage of its position close to the sea, the Beau Soleil had central heating, a vital feature missing from any of the houses he had lived in before. You can go to the South of France in search of light in the winter, but there are many days on which anyone who is also looking for warmth will be disappointed.

Central heating was a major concession on his part. Only a few years before, he had been sarcastic about those who turned up the radiator, glanced at the thermometer and said, 'We're just a bit below the level in here', before returning to their newspaper. For them, he had felt, there was no vivid relationship with the living universe; they had allowed technology to intervene between themselves and physical reality, numbing and atrophying their senses. What had pleased him about New, and more particularly Old Mexico was that there the reality of life appeared more in evidence, even if that reality often turned out to be harsh and cruel. He had lived in what he had thought was a real world until 1914 but had been deeply disillusioned by all that followed the outbreak of the Great War. His difficulties then had taught him that human nature was nowhere near as pleasant as he had believed and in Mexico he felt he learned that the same was true of Nature herself. Central heating was a minor feature in the occlusion of this second lesson and he disapproved of it, feeling that it was always better to be in contact with a true state of affairs: an open fire perhaps, but not a radiator. Yet failing health is often destructive of principles. In the Beau Soleil he could be comfortable with a minimum of effort, or at least his perpetual discomfort was not increased by being cold. The house was too small to accommodate all but the most intimate of his many visitors but he was able to direct them to the Beau Rivage, fulfilling the duties of hospitality by generously settling the bills of the poorer ones who stayed there.

Two people who stayed at the Beau Rivage at their own expense rather than his were Earl and Achsah Brewster, an American couple with a modest private income who preferred to live away from their native country. He had met the Brewsters when he visited Capri after the war and an initial bond was strengthened when it turned out that the Fontana Vecchia was the same villa in which they had spent their honeymoon. The Brewsters were interested in art and Eastern philosophies and had persuaded him to spend six weeks with them in Sri Lanka where the climate and the food had made him very ill. They themselves were vegetarians to the dismay of the proprietor of the Beau Rivage who asked him how people could choose to eat like that, 'C'est manger sans vouloir manger, n'est-ce pas?' But he liked them very much and it was at his request they had come to Bandol. They were only staying at the hotel while they looked for a house to rent in the neighbourhood where they could in some very small part fulfil his dream of a community of like-minded souls who would live in close proximity, isolated as much as possible from the modern world with its competition, pursuit of 'pleasure', and money-making: 'it is always my idea', he had once said, 'that a few people by being together should bring to pass a new earth and a new heaven.' In the meantime Earl Brewster was free to walk regularly over to the Beau Soleil and massage his friend's whole body with special medicinal oils.

Belief in the efficacy of body massage was a manifestation of Brewster's interest in yoga but at the sanatorium in Davos which Thomas Mann describes in *The Magic Mountain*, the young hero Hans Castorp receives daily massage as part of the treatment for tuberculosis. Brewster reported that the body he handled seemed to him like that of the crucified Jesus. This was a comparison which had followed its subject for much of his life: in Hertfordshire, during the war, the local boys had called him a 'walking Jesus' and later, in the streets of Oaxaca, their Mexican equivalents, responding to the reddish beard and gaunt frame, had murmured 'Cristos, Cristos' as he went by. He was quite a tall man for his time: 5′ 9″ according to one of his passports, but slight. Asking friends in Florence to find him a replica of a light blue jacket he had particularly enjoyed wearing, he gave his width across the shoulders, from armpit to armpit, as 15½ inches. A more comprehensive view of his physique was provided by his friend Knud Merrild after they had both sat naked in some hot springs near his New Mexican ranch in the mid-1920s. Merrild was a champion swimmer who had represented

Denmark in the Olympic Games and was able to take an expert view. 'I would not call him skinny', he wrote, 'but rather say he was slim with thin legs like the Archbishop of Canterbury, or like most Englishmen, but otherwise a well-proportioned body, harmonious in its slimness.' There is a puzzle here as to when Merrild had previously sat in a hot spring with a naked Archbishop, but the kind of physique he is describing is recognizable enough. It is not one which easily puts on much weight but by now the emaciation was alarming. 'I only weigh something over six stones', he was to say in February 1930, '—and even in the spring I was over seven, nearly eight.' As he tried to restore some vitality to his friend's body with his massages, Brewster thought it 'terrifying in its meagreness'.

From her first meeting with him, his wife had been a great admirer of his legs and it is striking how often in his fiction his male protagonists are praised for this part of their anatomy. Quick, alive, vital, the leg is a metonymy for animal vigour and sexual prowess. But now she lamented that her husband's legs had become 'so thin, so thin'. For several years they had slept in separate rooms whenever their circumstances made that possible. If he now asked her to sleep with him it was because in the past her simple presence by his side had brought him ease and comfort. The experiment was not a success. She felt that his awareness of her healthy body next to his had only increased his discomfort and concluded sadly that she could do nothing more for him. When Barbara Weekley, or Barby as she was always called, the younger of her two daughters from her previous marriage, came across him in the garden of the Beau Soleil, covered in rugs and with a grey, drawn expression on his face, he told her sadly: 'Your mother is repelled by the death in me.'

2

Tuberculosis

D H. Lawrence died on 2 March 1930. In that year there were 60,000 registered deaths from tuberculosis in France and 50,000 in Great Britain. As a disease of the lungs, tuberculosis was by far the biggest and most consistent killer in Western Europe throughout the nineteenth and the first half of the twentieth centuries. Grim though the figures for 1930 were, they represented a decline. Improved living conditions and more expert palliative care meant that the graph was heading slowly down so that it later became possible to argue that its steep descent in the 1950s and 1960s, after the introduction of streptomycin and other associated drugs, was not the miracle it must have seemed at the time, and that the comparative insignificance to which tuberculosis was eventually reduced in the latter half of the twentieth century (before the appearance of HIV/Aids and then of a strain of the disease resistant to antibiotics) was something which would have happened *anyway*. That is a doubtful proposition but, even it were true, it could hardly lessen our sense of the impact that streptomycin must have had when it first appeared. Here at last was something which could fairly be described as a cure for tuberculosis whereas nearly all previous treatments represented more or less efficacious methods of waiting for it to go away.

So prevalent was tuberculosis in the England of Lawrence's time that you would be bound to know many people affected by it. He was born on 11 September 1885 in a small terraced house on a street which runs steeply downhill from the high street in Eastwood, not many miles from Nottingham. But the family was upwardly mobile. It is true that their first move was further downhill, to a house which was bigger and could better accommodate a growing family. Mrs Lawrence did not like the new neighbourhood and, as her children became older and some of them began to work, she was able to move back up the hill to a house which had a bay window and was in a new development referred to by the locals as 'piano row'. The Lawrences then moved again, to a similar house but one which this time had the virtue of being semi-detached. Their landlord was called Tom Cooper and lived next door. He had five daughters and a wife who in 1904 died of tuberculosis at the age of 55. Twenty years later four of these daughters were dead from the same disease and the fifth, Gertie, was being treated for it. An indication of the closeness of the Lawrence and Cooper families is that in 1919 Gertie went to live with Lawrence's favourite sister, Ada; and he himself wrote to her frequently, trying to keep up her spirits and offering advice on the various treatments she endured.

Lawrence would have seen around him enough cases like the Coopers' to reject the myth, most commonly associated by the English with Keats, that tuberculosis chiefly afflicted people of an artistic or literary temperament; yet he had good reason also to be aware that those with such temperaments were by no means immune. In the early part of the First World War he was an occasional member of the group of anti-war intellectuals and artists which Lady Ottoline Morrell would gather together at Garsington, her country house in Oxfordshire. A more frequent visitor there was the painter Mark Gertler. Lawrence was an unusual figure among Lady Ottoline's friends because his background was working class but Gertler was even more unusual in that his parents were Polish Jews who had settled in London's East End where their gifted son was brought up in crowded and impoverished surroundings. In 1920 he was found to have tuberculosis and sent to a sanatorium near Aberdeen. This was the same institution in which Somerset Maugham had been treated three years earlier and it specialized in a fresh air treatment which had been pioneered in Germany. What this chiefly comprised, Maugham suggests in the short story he based on his stay there, was a patient breathing in as much cold Scottish air as possible while the body was wrapped in rugs or covered in furs. Gertler recovered but the disease reappeared five years later. This time he was sent to a sanatorium which was acquiring a reputation for being the best in England, and where Gertie Cooper spent some time, the Mundesley in Norfolk. Again he recovered. The question of quite how complete his recovery was is complicated by the fact that Gertler committed suicide in 1939, when he was 48.

Gertler's case and, more especially, that of Somerset Maugham (who lived into his nineties), show that tuberculosis was not necessarily fatal although one survey has indicated that of all the people who received sanatorium treatment in 1914, 80 per cent were dead six years later. Katherine Mansfield was a less fortunate and closer friend of Lawrence's than Gertler, and another occasional member of the Garsington set. When at the end of 1917 she was told that she had a spot on one of her lungs she went off to Bandol for rest and recuperation and thereafter did all she could to get better. Her efforts included putting herself in the hands of a dubious Russian doctor who claimed that he could eradicate her disease by bombarding the spleen with X-rays; and it was largely because of the propaganda of another Russian, Pyotr Uspensky, that she ended her days at the Institute for the Harmonious Development of Man run by Georges Gurdjieff. There was always something potentially contradictory in the advice tubercular patients were likely to receive. They were often advised to avoid the cold of the English climate by moving to towns on the French or Italian Riviera while, at the same time, cold mountain air was highly recommended. Gurdjieff's Institute was in Fontainebleau, near Paris, and a long way from either the Mediterranean or the mountains. The town is low in altitude and does not have a particularly mild climate but then the Institute was not a sanatorium but rather a commune where disciples of its charismatic leader could forge a new way of living which, it was supposed, would bring better health in its train. All who went there were given manual tasks and made to live in quite primitive conditions, making their own beds and washing in cold water. The principal concession made to Mansfield's state was that she was told to sit on a platform above a cowshed, the rising steam from which was thought by peasants in Russia to have a beneficial effect on those with her disease. When her husband Middleton Murry went to see her in January 1923 an artery in one of her diseased lungs ruptured and blood poured from her mouth. By the time expert help was on hand she was dead, perhaps because she had choked on her own blood, although the commonest terminal event in tuberculosis was an accumulation of sputum in the larynx which the patient became too weak to cough up. In the usual and probably accurate account, Murry witnessed her death but Lawrence (who had quarrelled with him) chose to believe a different story. He had heard that when Mansfield was told her husband was in the vicinity, she exclaimed 'Keep that bugger away from me' and had her fatal haemorrhage before he entered her room.

It has been suggested that it was Lawrence who infected Mansfield with tuberculosis. This would have been in 1916 when he had persuaded her and Murry to come and live close by himself and his wife Frieda in Cornwall, and the two couples were in constant communication. Tuberculosis is chiefly spread by droplets of sputum when the infected person coughs in the presence of others, with repeated close contact an important factor. It is possible then that Lawrence was the culprit but quite how far tuberculosis is infectious is a complicated subject. This is in part because almost everyone in England during the years of its dominance could be said to have had it in the sense that the overwhelming majority would have suffered a primary infection during childhood and continued to harbour the bacterium in a dormant form. At the same time, they would have acquired an immunity against the development of the disease which would only be damaged later where there was some genetic predisposition (and the history of families like the Coopers suggest that genetic factors were important), or when they were in a particularly run-down and enfeebled state. Mansfield was frequently ill in the period leading up to 1916 and may have contracted tuberculosis from Lawrence but, given its ubiquity, there were plenty of other occasions when she could have picked it up. To be sure that he was the source, we would have to know not merely that he was already tubercular in 1916, but that his disease was then in an active phase. The surviving evidence casts some doubt on at least the second of these propositions.

In her last years, Mansfield was subject to outbursts of uncontrollable rage which she identified as one of the symptoms of her tuberculosis. It was her memory of Lawrence's similar outbursts in 1916 which later convinced her that he must already have been suffering then from the disease which was only to be diagnosed in her a year later. But rage, moments of frenzy when he became oblivious of his environment and seemed possessed by some demon of blind anger, was characteristic of Lawrence from his early youth, well before he knew Mansfield, so that to interpret it as a symptom would be to stretch the onset of his tuberculosis a long way back. The first observation on his health came when his mother was pushing him in a pram while he was still a baby and was met in the street by an Eastwood neighbour, Willie Hopkin. She sometimes wondered, Mrs Lawrence told Hopkin, whether she would ever be able to raise such a delicate child. Confirmation that he was delicate and often ill comes from the fact that he did not attend school regularly until he was 7. In 1901, when he was 16, he fell seriously ill with pneumonia and was thought to be in danger of dying. What helped to pull him through was the devoted nursing of Mrs Lawrence who was rescued by the illness of this son from the emotional torpor into which the recent death of an older one, Ernest, had thrown her. It was now that Lawrence solidified that intense bond with his mother which he was later to characterize as distorting and unhealthy. In 1911 he was again gravely ill with pneumonia although this time, with his mother dead, it was his sister Ada who was his principal nurse. He was told as he began to recover that he must not go back to his job as a schoolteacher because he was 'threatened with consumption'. This was a common category of the time, so much so that in France there was a special word, the *preventorium,* which designated institutions where those who fell into it might be sent. Yet it was also as he was recovering that Lawrence had the all-important sputum test with samples of his saliva being taken to a laboratory where well-tried methods were employed to detect in it the tubercular bacillus. As his sister reported with some relief in December 1911, the test was negative. 'The expectoration was very satisfactory,' Ada said, 'No germs were discovered.'

David Garnett, who regarded Lawrence as something of a lower-class cad in his treatment of a wife whose maiden name had been von Richthofen, claimed to have once spotted in 1913 'one of Frieda's handkerchiefs, marked with a coronet in the corner, crumpled in Lawrence's hand, after a fit of coughing and spotted with bright arterial blood'. This gave him, he explained, a new tenderness for Lawrence and readiness to forgive his bad moods. But there is no other suggestion of his having tuberculosis at this time, or in the five years of the war. In 1915, shortly before the Murrys came down to join him in Cornwall, he was examined by a doctor friend who clearly did not believe he was tubercular; in 1917 he had himself thoroughly inspected in London and returned to Cornwall reassured; and during the whole period of the war he was obliged to undergo several medical inspections, none of which led to a positive diagnosis. As far as any real knowledge of his tuberculosis is concerned, therefore, the crucial phase begins in 1924 when he and Frieda were living on the ranch in New Mexico. At the beginning of August in that year Lawrence began to spit a good deal of bright red blood. The description comes from his friend Dorothy Brett, who was living with the Lawrences at the time and who, having helped to nurse Katherine Mansfield, knew that a bright red colour was the distinctive sign of a pulmonary haemorrhage rather than any other kind of bleeding from the mouth. Yet when the local doctor came he said that Lawrence's lungs were strong and all that was troubling him was a little bronchial trouble. Six months later, when he and Frieda were living in the small Mexican town of Oaxaca, he fell dangerously ill. His symptoms this time appeared to have little to do with his chest but rather his bowels and he himself concluded that he was suffering from malaria contracted when he was with the Brewsters in Sri Lanka. Whatever the problem, it was sufficiently serious to make him feel he might die but, with Frieda's help, he struggled to Mexico City and put himself in the hands of doctors there. Their examination included a chest X-ray and a sputum test, the combined result of which showed that Lawrence's luck had run out and one of his lungs was affected with tuberculosis. It was only therefore in March 1925 that we can be sure Lawrence might have been a danger to others although Frieda never suffered any ill effects. According to a textbook of the time, the likelihood of someone being infected by a sick partner was only slightly higher than the chances of developing tuberculosis in the population as a whole, and the difference could be attributed to the stress and fatigue associated with nursing the sick or dying.

There is a cruel irony in the situation of all those who suffered from tuberculosis between the 1880s and the 1950s. In 1882 Robert

Koch had announced his discovery of the bacillus which was at the root of the trouble and thereafter increasingly reliable tests were developed for detecting it in the sputum. Backed up by the emerging science of radiography, these made diagnosis more and more certain. When R. L. Stevenson or H. G. Wells coughed a lot, ran high temperatures, brought up large amounts of phlegm, and suffered night sweats or the occasional haemorrhage, there was a strong suspicion they were tubercular but no way of being sure. By Lawrence's time you did not need a post-mortem to tell. Yet knowing tuberculosis was present did not mean there was a great deal to be done. Sensible treatment consisted in an ingenious variety of methods for encouraging the body to resist the disease and cure itself. Only with the discovery of streptomycin in 1944 did the doctors have a non-surgical weapon which allowed them to be anything more than defensive. For seventy years therefore they knew the cause without having any safe and sure means of eradicating it.

It is natural to feel regret that the discovery and development of an effective drug therapy came too late to help Mansfield and Lawrence and this kind of regret will be keener in the case of George Orwell whose tubercular condition began to worsen dramatically in the late 1940s. Orwell was fortunate in having in David Astor a rich and influential friend who could write to the United States for a quantity of streptomycin at a time when it was still being tested by the British medical authorities and had not yet been officially approved. But when it was administered to Orwell he developed such a violent allergic reaction that it had to be discontinued. It would, in any case, be some time before it was realized that the drug needed to be combined with others for it to be lastingly rather than only temporarily effective. The circumstances of Orwell's death in 1950, when he was 46, have therefore something of the same poignancy as those of men who die in the last months or weeks of a war. In both cases, we are inclined to feel that just a little more time would have seen them through and it is obviously true that had Orwell fallen ill just a little later, then he might have lived many more years and written many more books.

That these are natural thoughts and feelings does not prove that they are therefore wholly rational. Over the past hundred and fifty years there has been a steady progress in medical science. This means that anyone lying ill in the first half of the twentieth century could have felt that at least their treatment would be better than if they had found themselves in the same situation at any time during the century before. In his youth Lawrence would take trips to Newstead Abbey, which is only a few miles from Eastwood and is where Byron spent some of his boyhood. The two Nottinghamshire writers came from opposite ends of the social spectrum but were like each other in the outrage they caused to conventional English opinion and their decision to spend the latter part of their lives in voluntary exile. Byron died at the age of 36 in Greece of what is now thought to have been uraemic poisoning. His doctors could do nothing about that but they destroyed any hope his system might have had of resisting his illness by administering strong purgatives and by bleeding him continuously. Byron disapproved of bleeding, claiming that more people had been killed by the lancet than the lance, but he became too weak to prevent his doctors constantly applying their leeches and opening his veins. Doctors in Lawrence's time had scarcely more power over tuberculosis than Bryon's had over his uraemic poisoning, but they understood much better the nature of their patients' diseases and, with notable exceptions like the Russian who bombarded Mansfield's spleen with X-rays, were unlikely in their ministrations to do more harm than good. In that sense, Lawrence was fortunate to be ill in 1930 but in another he was unlucky not to have had the benefit of treatments which were developed twenty-five years later: had he lived to be 75 he would have been able to speak up for himself at the *Lady Chatterley* trial. What makes the regret that he did not have that benefit irrational is the position that we are all fated to occupy on the rising graph of progress in medical science. There are contingent factors which can affect our chances of survival: falling ill at the wrong time and in the wrong place, misdiagnosis, a visit to the wrong doctor. But in the more general view we all die too soon with discoveries which would allow us to survive just around the corner. On this topic, the Romanian poet Marin Sorescu has expressed a very natural thought in a poem most of the poetry of which seems to have been unavoidably lost in translation:

> When the cure for a disease is discovered
> Those who have died of the illness
> Ought to rise again
> And go on living
> All the rest of their days
> Until they fall sick with another disease
> Whose cure has not yet been discovered.

It seems clear that a writer well known for his irony is here pointing out that, on the assumption that we all have to die *of* something, fairness for all would mean immortality for the same number.

3

Denial

There are moments in the lives of many people when doctors feel obliged to give them bad news. No very clear protocols exist about how to respond to this news, nor indeed about how to impart it. For most of the years of its terrifying dominance the burden of cure in tuberculosis lay heavily on the patient, and doctors were therefore well aware of the importance of psychological factors. The chief doctor at the Mundesley sanatorium in the late 1920s and early 1930s was Andrew Morland. In his handbook entitled *Pulmonary Tuberculosis in General Practice,* published in 1932, Morland wrote: 'Hope is certainly a great stimulant, and as few cases are hopeless from the start, the doctor should give the patient the benefit of the doubt and confidently assume that eventual recovery will occur.'

From the Mundesley, Morland eventually moved to University College Hospital in London and it was there that he treated George Orwell, encouraging him to believe that, although he would need to live the rest of his life as a chronic invalid, he was in no immediate danger. What Morland said must have influenced Orwell's decision to marry. The wedding took place in a private room of the hospital on 13 October 1949 and just over three months later Orwell died from a pulmonary haemorrhage in that same room. Quite when a tubercular patient might suffer a haemorrhage was impossible to predict and as a general rule prognosis in tuberculosis was never easy. It was well known that patients whose cases seemed hopeless sometimes made startling recoveries while others, who appeared to be only mildly affected, were dead in a few weeks. There was nevertheless the danger in being optimistic of telling people what they wanted to hear rather than what, for practical as well as psychological reasons, they might need to know.

The doctors whom Lawrence saw in Mexico City in 1925 were from the American Hospital and could not be accused of lack of directness or a misleading optimism. They said that he had tuberculosis 'in the third degree' and were not sanguine about his chances of survival. These were judgements communicated in the first instance to Frieda, but she remembered returning to the hotel room where she and her husband were staying and finding someone she calls the 'analyst doctor' already there. 'Mr Lawrence has tuberculosis' this doctor announced to her rather brutally and that the person being spoken about overheard is evident from Frieda's associated memory of her husband then looking at her 'with unforgettable eyes'.

Lawrence's response to his bad news seems at first an obvious case of what it is now fashionable to call denial: that same phenomenon which leads alcoholics to insist they do not drink immoderately and to avoid therefore the first step which could lead to their recovery. On only one subsequent occasion in the five remaining years of his life did Lawrence use the word tubercular in relation to himself, and that was little more than a fortnight before he died. What he otherwise always maintained was that it was his 'bronchials' which gave him trouble, not his lungs, repeating this distinction like a mantra as if to protect himself from the fate of people like Gertie Cooper or Katherine Mansfield. As late as November 1929 he told Mark Gertler, 'My bronchials are really awful. It's not the lungs,' but this was a claim he had made very many times before. The impression he gives is of someone who seeks to wish away the threat of tuberculosis by refusing to acknowledge it has any relevance to himself.

That impression may be largely accurate but it is complicated by a few remarks Lawrence made towards the end of his life. In the summer of 1929 he was in Baden-Baden, on a visit to his mother-in-law, and arranged to see a doctor there. The doctor says, he reported to his friend Giuseppe Orioli on 7 August, that 'the lung is better', and three days later he told the same correspondent that 'my lung is healed, but my bronchials and asthma only a little better', asthma being the term he had settled on for his constant breathlessness. Here at least was an indirect admission that there had once been something wrong with his lungs. Three weeks before he died his chest was X-rayed and on 12 February 1930 he told Maria Huxley that 'the lung has moved very little since Mexico, in five years'. He could hardly have offered this comparison had he not known a good deal about the Mexico City X-ray, or even carried a copy with him. What his making of it suggests is that it was not so much the diagnosis of the Mexican doctors which he contested but their view of its implications. What he denied is that having something wrong with his lungs, or once having had something wrong with them, bore in any significant way on his steadily worsening state.

Denial can be taken as part of the pathology of a certain condition or it can be related to character: did Lawrence lack the courage and honesty to face up to the truth? This last possibility seems important because of the searing emotional honesty Lawrence often displayed in other aspects of his life, and in his work. Part of the initial impact of novels like *The Rainbow* or *Women in Love* lay in their author's evident willingness to discover and acknowledge in himself feelings which in the majority of his readers were either ignored or repressed. How could the man who wrote these works shy away from the truth of his own condition? Even if he had been in a position to demonstrate that the *major* reason for his increasingly lamentable state was the acute bronchitis of someone who had suffered from chest complaints all his life, should he not have acknowledged openly the tuberculosis in his lungs as a vital contributory cause so that steps could be taken to deal with it?

There were many severe psychological problems associated with admitting you had tuberculosis in Lawrence's time but also several practical ones. Official statistics were dismaying, but they were probably less so than they might have been because of a reluctance on the part of some to report tubercular cases to the authorities. These would be doctors in the poorer sections of a community who understood fully, not only the moral stigma attached to the disease, but also the consequences which identifying it would have on a patient's future employment prospects. A man in his thirties whose lungs were affected might have ten or more years to live, with times during those years when he was quite well; but if he had to provide for a family in that period, being labelled tubercular would hardly help. Because tuberculosis was frequently the cause of lingering rather than sudden death, it illustrates well the unfairness of illnesses, taking away easy physical well-being while at the same time loading the weakened frame with extra weights in the battle of life.

The practical disadvantages of having tuberculosis were made apparent to Lawrence almost immediately after the diagnosis in Mexico City. He had planned to take the boat to England and convalesce somewhere on the South Coast. But one doctor had told Frieda that his only hope was a period of rest at high altitude and the Lawrences therefore decided to go back to their ranch in the mountains above Taos. Returning there meant re-entering the United States whose government had recently passed legislation aimed at preventing anyone with tuberculosis from coming into the country. Despite using rouge to disguise the unhealthy pallor of his cheeks, Lawrence was stopped at the border in El Paso and subjected to a humiliating medical inspection. Only after many hours, and when strings had been pulled in various consulates, was he let through.

The visa he was finally given in El Paso allowed him to get back to the ranch (which had been a gift to Frieda from Mabel Dodge Luhan, a rich American admirer of her husband), but it was valid for only six months. When therefore he left the United States in September 1925 he ought to have recognized he could never return. Yet because he had after all recovered at the ranch, he often talked later of going back there. He would say that what deterred him were possible immigration difficulties without ever making clear to friends, and perhaps to himself, what those difficulties were. Near the end of his life, having failed to get well in so many different places in Europe, Taos loomed ever larger, a forlorn hope; and he sent his stepdaughter Barby to enquire about visas. But the doctor who examined him at this time, and who happened to be Andrew Morland, felt that even if the immigration difficulties could be overcome, Lawrence was far too weak to survive the journey.

Lawrence's problems with the American immigration service suggest that it was not always expedient to admit to having tuberculosis; but if expediency was in fact one of the reasons for the attitude he adopted towards his illness, there were many others. One of these was a distrust of doctors in so far as they were representatives of modern, scientific medicine, as the 'analyst' in Mexico City certainly was. Like many of his contemporaries, Lawrence resented the dominant position science was beginning to assume in Western culture and in particular its presumption to be able to explain everything, then or at some future date. His hostility could lead him into anti-rationalist absurdities, sometimes expressed bluntly and sometimes wittily as when, in *Fantasia of the Unconscious*, he says that to assume mind evolved from matter is like taking a cart, spraying it with white wine, and then expecting to see it groan and writhe until a horse lay panting between the shafts. He was sceptical of evolutionary theory in its then current, vulgarized forms (as if my ancestors, he complained, had no more up their sleeve than 'just the marvel of the unborn me'), and he refused to accept any version of our origins which did not leave him, as he puts it, intuitively and instinctively convinced. This was part of a general view which helped determine his attitude to his own condition. Since he could not feel the spots on his lung which the X-ray revealed, or since any trouble they gave him was initially masked by more obvious difficulties emanating from his bronchial tubes, why should he believe a machine rather than what his own body told him?

In the introduction to his 1932 edition of Lawrence's letters, Aldous Huxley left a highly influential if somewhat simplified account of his friend's approach to science. It was a topic on which they had often had violent arguments, he wrote, and he remembered how during one of these, which centred on evolution, he had simply asked Lawrence to consider the evidence. According to Huxley, Lawrence replied that evidence meant nothing to him unless he could feel convinced *here*, and he laid his hand on his solar plexus. When it came to questions of health, Huxley found this attitude painfully exasperating. In March 1929, at the end of his first stay in Bandol, Lawrence travelled up to Paris in order to arrange for the publication of a cheap, popular edition of *Lady Chatterley's Lover*. Without Frieda, who had gone to visit her mother (and her Italian lover), he arranged to stay with Aldous and Maria Huxley in the Paris suburb of Suresnes. The Huxleys were appalled by his state and, profiting from the greater vulnerability he felt without Frieda's presence, they persuaded him to see a doctor. This doctor told Maria that, from listening to Lawrence's chest, he suspected that one lung was already gone and that the other was badly affected and he made an appointment for an X-ray. When, however, the time came for the appointment, Lawrence refused to keep it and, with Frieda once more by his side, quickly retreated to the warmer south. For Aldous this was the behaviour of someone who simply did not want to know how ill he was but Lawrence himself later wrote one of his little poems, or 'pansies' as he called them, in which he claimed to have detected in the 'scientific doctor' he saw in Paris 'a lust...to wreak his so-called science on me | and reduce me to the level of a thing'.

'The Scientific Doctor' was written in the summer of 1929 at around the same time as a poem called 'Healing' in which Lawrence asked himself why he was so ill. The answer he gave was certainly not the bacterium Koch had discovered in 1882. If he was ill, he decided, it was not because his mechanism was working wrongly since 'a mechanism, an assembly of various sections' is what he had never been. The cause of his difficulties was rather a series of 'wounds to the soul, to the deep emotional self' and the only cure lay in 'long, difficult repentance, realisation of life's mistake'. This is a resolutely psychosomatic view of illness not surprising in someone who refused to believe that matter preceded mind. But if disease had its origin in states of mind and feeling it followed, as 'Healing' suggests, that it could sometimes be defeated by an alteration in those states. This was always Lawrence's view and it has much to recommend it although on occasions his belief in the power of mind over matter can seem obscurantist, prejudiced, and strident. On 10 December 1918, for example, he wrote a letter to Katherine Mansfield immediately after having returned from Ripley in Derbyshire where he had found one of Gertie Cooper's sisters 'just on the point of dying' of tuberculosis (she was buried a fortnight later). To the already ailing Mansfield he insisted: 'Katherine, *on ne meurt pas* . . . Be damned and be blasted everything, and let the bloody world come to its end. But one does not die. *Jamais.*' The startling vehemence of these remarks has affinities with the account in Samuel Richardson's novel *Clarissa* of the death of the wicked old brothel-keeper Mrs Sinclair who has broken her leg and, because mortification has set in, is told by Belford that she will certainly die:

> *Die*, did you say, sir? *Die!* I *will not*, I *cannot* die! I know not *how* to die! *Die*, sir! And *must* I then die? Leave this world? I cannot bear it! And who brought *you* hither, sir (her eyes striking fire at me), to tell me I must *die*, sir? I cannot, I will not leave this world.

Lawrence's defiance was of course principally adopted on Mansfield's behalf rather than his own and it was probably designed to buck her up, to counter a tendency he may have felt she had, not to the Christian resignation Richardson's narrative advocates, but to defeatism and apathy. Yet when he came to rely on it for his own purposes, it would sometimes demonstrate how thin the dividing line can be between a mindless refusal to face up to the truth and that 'positive frame of mind' which doctors always insist is so vital in defeating disease.

Katherine Mansfield was someone of whom Lawrence was particularly fond but the fondness meant that his fallings-out with her were particularly vitriolic. The last of them led to what is perhaps the most discreditable episode of his career: the letter from early 1920 in which he told her 'you revolt me stewing in your consumption'. Attempts have been made to palliate the offensiveness of this sentence by suggesting that it should be read with an emphasis on the 'your', and that Lawrence was implicitly comparing Mansfield's attitude to tuberculosis with his own. But 1920 is long before he had been told he was tubercular so that it seems more likely that he is expressing a general contempt for any surrender to illness. Our diseases might win out in the end—he knew very well that, sooner or later, one does in fact die—but in the meantime the last thing to do was 'stew' in them. What may be surfacing here also, however, is a prejudice which he had aired as long ago as 1908 when he first read *The Shropshire Lad* and complained that its author, A. E. Housman, could 'only sing the stale tale of the bankruptcy of life'. 'I believe he comes of a consumptive family', he then said, 'I believe he himself is consumptive. Bah!' In someone who had experienced problems with his chest from a very early age, stigmatizing consumptives may have been a private method for warding off evil similar in unconscious intention to his insistence to a friend in 1913 that although his lungs were 'crocky', he was 'not consumptive, the type, as they say. I am not really afraid of consumption,' he went on, 'I don't know why—I don't think I shall ever die of *that*.'

If Lawrence's remarks on Housman, and his denial that he himself was the consumptive type, were meant to ward off evil and death from tuberculosis, if they were (that is) what Freud called apotropaic, then it is possible to make a case for thinking they succeeded. Medical diagnosis of figures from the past increases in difficulty the longer it is since they died. Being certain of what Byron was suffering from in Messolonghi in 1824 is impossible (uraemic poisoning is only one medical authority's recent, highly educated guess), and it is still hard to be sure of the precise reasons for Lawrence's death in 1930. It could be claimed that the recurrent bouts of bronchitis to which he had always been prone so weakened his constitution that they ought to be cited as the principal cause. In the last week of his life he was reported as having developed pleurisy or an inflammation of the coverings of the lungs. It is difficult to tell whether this should be regarded as a fresh, separate illness or merely a further manifestation of the tuberculosis from which he was undoubtedly then suffering. Yet even if, technically speaking, his prediction was right and '*that*' disease was not the immediate cause of his death, what one can say with confidence is that it certainly did not help.

4

The Sanatorium

By denying that he had tuberculosis, or that he was seriously affected by it, Lawrence turned his back on what in his time was thought to be the most effective treatment: an extended stay in a sanatorium. The vogue for sanatoria had begun in the 1860s and spread rapidly throughout Europe. The principal idea was to remove patients from the cares and stresses of their daily existence and impose on them a strict regime of relaxation, over-feeding, gentle exercise, and the breathing in of uncontaminated air. Published in 1924, Thomas Mann's *The Magic Mountain* gives a memorable picture of sanatorium life and helped to win him the Nobel Prize; but there is another vivid account in *The Rack* by Derek Lindsay, whose pseudonym was A. E. Ellis. *The Rack*, which was published in 1958, deals with the years after the Second World War and shows that the need for sanatoria diminished gradually rather than vanishing as soon as streptomycin and other effective drugs came into use. It is a novel which has neither the philosophical breadth, the wit, nor the variety of characterization of *The Magic Mountain* but, as far as the treatment of tuberculosis is concerned, it is in many ways more detailed and inward. A likely reason for this is that Lindsay was himself a patient in a sanatorium in France whereas much of Mann's information came from visiting his wife when she was obliged to spend some time at an expensive sanatorium in Switzerland.

The experience of Mark Gertler illustrates some of the drawbacks of the sanatorium for a person in Lawrence's position, and for someone of his temperament. Patients usually began their stay with a period of complete bed rest when they were not allowed to do anything apart from eat, drink, and lie on balconies inhaling pure air. There would during this time, that is, have been no writing for Lawrence just as there was no painting for Gertler, who found the boredom excruciating and who was also nauseated by the endless round of meals. After this initial period, which could sometimes last many months, patients were allowed to get up and prescribed regular hours of gentle and graduated outdoor exercise. The whole process of cure or rehabilitation could be very lengthy and therefore very expensive. There were in Britain cheap or sometimes free sanatoria run by charities or the public authorities but these tended to be at the prison-camp end of the market rather than that of Mann's five-star hotel. The sanatorium in Scotland cost Gertler £45 each month (half of Lawrence's annual salary when he had begun work as a teacher), and he was there for more than half a year. The Mundesley was dearer, the most expensive sanatorium in England. In Gertler's case the cost was largely borne by the members of his family who were not at all rich. Neither of course were those of Lawrence's family. During the war years, after *The Rainbow* had been banned and he found it impossible to find outlets for his work, Lawrence was often desperately poor and driven at times to accept help from family members, Ada in particular. In ways which he found deeply humiliating, he was also occasionally reliant on the charity of well-disposed individuals or of public bodies such as the Royal Literary Fund. By the time of the diagnosis in Mexico City his fortunes were much improved thanks in large part to success in the American market, and not a little to a failed attempt by the New York Society for the Suppression of Vice to have *Women in Love* banned. But he was still far from well off and the unpaid royalties which resulted from the business failure of his American publisher, Thomas Seltzer, made it seem unlikely that he ever would be. An extended stay in a sanatorium would almost certainly have thrown a very proud man back once again on the charity of others, have made him once again a 'charity boy of literature' as he had once bitterly described himself. The trouble with sanatoria for people like Gertler and Lawrence, as well as of course for thousands of others, was that they proscribed the means of earning money while simultaneously increasing a need for it.

Another drawback of life in a sanatorium as far as Lawrence was concerned is that it encouraged patients to treat themselves like the invalids they undoubtedly were. As a way of forcing them to take an interest in their own health, they were made to record their own temperatures every morning and evening, keeping the thermometer in the mouth for a minimum of seven minutes. Temperature-taking was important because it could suggest whether the tuberculosis bacterium was still active and both Mann and Lindsay paint a lively picture of what an important ritual it became with patients elated by the slightest drop or depressed by any rise. It was after his first stay in a sanatorium that Gertler began keeping a health journal in which he recorded his temperature regularly and kept an eye on his weight. From then on he also made sure that he drank a pint and a half of milk every day, strictly controlled his hours of work, and took daily walks. That is to say, he acknowledged, as life in the sanatorium had taught him to, that he was not like other, healthy people and needed to keep a close watch on himself.

This was sensible behaviour but a problem for Lawrence in adopting it could be summed up economically, if not *entirely* fairly, in the one word Frieda. Had he married his first girlfriend Jessie Chambers, or Louie Burrows, the girl to whom he became engaged just before his mother's death in December 1910, he would have had no difficulty in declaring himself an invalid and committing himself to their tender care. They would have been only too pleased to mother him. But mothering was not in Frieda's line and nor was it something Lawrence wanted, keen as he had been to escape the influence of his own mother and alert as he always was to the subtle perversions it could engender in relationships between those of a similar age. In *Lady Chatterley's Lover* Sir Clifford Chatterley, badly wounded during the war, finds a substitute mother in his nurse Mrs Bolton but his wife abandons him. There is a stern Nietzschean morality in Lawrence's treatment of this situation which insists that no injuries on the scale Clifford suffers them are without corresponding psychological impairment and that therefore their victims necessarily become a threat to the healthy and undamaged. In Nietzsche's view, the weak are inclined to prey on the strong by exploiting the latter's feelings of sympathy and guilt, or their sense of duty. But this is immoral because, as he writes in *The Genealogy of Morals*, 'Our first rule on this earth should be that the sick must not contaminate the healthy... The right to exist of the full-toned bell is a thousand times greater than that of the cracked, miscast one: it alone heralds the future of mankind.' Connie Chatterley is tied to Clifford by pity but the consequence is that, denied both sexual and emotional fulfilment, she becomes ill. The novel insists on her moral right to that fulfilment rather than on her Christian duty to her crippled and impotent husband. The way it is written suggests that Lawrence had always known, or at least always felt, that by adopting the life of an invalid he would forfeit any right to Frieda.

The usual course of treatment for tuberculosis in the sanatoria threatened the status of doctors in that their role was largely reduced to supervision: in its most common form, it did not give them the opportunity to fulfil the expectation of some patients that they should *do something*, and do it quickly. A frequent and dramatic addition to treatment was, however, the pneumothorax. The hero of *The Rack*, Paul Davenant, has a pneumothorax which is described in great detail. A needle is inserted between his fourth and fifth rib on his left side and air pumped into the space between the lung and the rib cage—the space known as the pleural cavity—with the result that the adjacent lung collapses. This procedure was performed under local anaesthetic and was relatively straightforward. There was a slight danger of careless doctors pushing the needle too far so that they punctured the lung and a rare, little understood phenomenon known as the 'pleural shock' which may have been the consequence of an air embolism and which could often be life-threatening. One of Mann's characters, Herr Ferge, has survived the pleural shock but been traumatized by it. He claims to remember the doctor trailing a needle over his pleura in order to find a suitable place to make an incision and 'let the gas in', a sensation he compares to being tickled, 'horribly, disgustingly tickled'. 'The pleura', he declares, 'is not anything that should be felt of; it does not want to be felt of and it ought not to be. It is taboo. It is covered up with flesh and put away once and for all; nobody and nothing ought to come near it.' The wholly exceptional nature of his case is, however, suggested in *The Magic Mountain* by the group of lively young girls that Hans Castorp meets on his first arrival in the sanatorium, one of whom is able to disconcert him by producing strange whistling noises directly from her chest. This is a side-effect of the pneumothorax which she and all her companions have had performed on them without any obvious ill effects. Together these young people have unofficially formed what they call the half-lung club. The principle of the pneumothorax was an extension of that on which sanatorium treatment in general was based. Collapsing a tubercular lung meant that it no longer had to work but could rest, and it was therefore hoped it would heal much quicker.

Although the pneumothorax was a relatively simple procedure it could of course only be performed on patients who had another lung which was healthy. A second disadvantage was that collapsed lungs begin to reinflate after only a week or two. Air had therefore to be reinjected at regular, briefly spaced intervals over a period which it was usually recommended should last years rather than months. A common sight in Lawrence's time was a queue of people who had been discharged from the sanatoria and who therefore lined up outside specially equipped dispensaries to have their 'refills'. Having continually to go back to a doctor in this way was inconvenient, but the patient could suffer something more than inconvenience if there were complications. In *The Rack* Derek Lindsay gives a harrowing description of a pneumothorax which goes wrong with tubercular infected pus filling Paul Davenant's chest and having then to be drained off via his sternum. A danger of even those 'pleural effusions' which did not signal infection was that they could lead to 'adhesions' with the parts of the pleura covering the lung and the rib cage sticking together so that the pleural cavity closed up and the pneumothorax could no longer be maintained. There was a tricky procedure for the surgical separation of these internal organs known as thoracoscopy which the unfortunate Paul is described as undergoing. When separation was not possible the lung could also be partially collapsed in a variety of other ways, the most common of which was a thoracoplasty, the removal of up to ten ribs. All of these procedures were usually carried out under local anaesthetic or, in the case of the injection of air-refills with a needle through the side, with no anaesthetic at all. But in his 1932 handbook Andrew Morland says of thoracoplasty that 'although the operation is commonly performed under local anaesthesia on the Continent, this is often a terrible strain', and he humanely recommends the use on the poor patient of a mixture of nitrous oxide and oxygen. In that way they would not hear the terrible cracking sound as the ribs were removed. An even more extreme procedure, which has nothing to do with collapse therapy, and which was already being practised in the 1920s, was the surgical removal of parts of an infected lung. In this case especially, but also in all the others described, the medical profession could hardly be accused of inactivity. Treatment of tuberculosis before streptomycin may largely have consisted in encouraging Nature to take a beneficial course, but there were ways of hurrying her along which gave to doctors a prominence they would not otherwise have had, and which the statistics of survival rates suggest was not wholly undeserved.

In that section of the British working class to which in his youth
Lawrence had so firmly belonged, there was a traditional distrust
of hospitals. Once they have you in, the feeling was, the only way
you will come out is feet first (a prejudice that has received some
support recently from news of the ravages in hospitals of the so-
called 'super-bugs'). A further, more legitimate reason for
apprehension was that once inside a hospital, which is what a
sanatorium was, the patient's power to accept or deny a certain
course of treatment was considerably weakened. Paul Davenant
suffers the whole range of surgical treatment for tuberculosis, with
the exception of lung removal, and the immediate consequences
are so painful and demoralizing that on two occasions he declares
firmly that he wants the doctors to leave him alone. But they
ignore his protests, convinced that what they are doing is for his
own good. He is powerless in their hands. This is a situation
Lawrence was always anxious to avoid and he must have
developed a pessimistic view of where a stay in a sanatorium
might eventually lead through his friendship with Gertie Cooper.
She was still living with his sister Ada when he made his final trip
to England in 1926. Everyone then was concerned about Gertie's
health and apprehensive that she was about to go the way of her
four sisters. Incongruously enough, Lawrence declared that she
had 'delayed too long' in seeking professional help and anxiously
discussed her case with both Gertler and Koteliansky, a Russian
émigré whom he had known since before the war. He pressed his
sister to have Gertie properly examined in Nottingham with those
same X-rays and sputum tests which, two years later in Paris,
he would be so anxious to avoid. When the results came through
he sent a knowledgeable report to Koteliansky, told him that there

was a new, active lesion on the top of the left lung, and made arrangements for Gertie to go to the Mundesley (there was money in her family). In view of his own recent history, this impatient concern to have Gertie properly looked after, and the degree of expertise he showed in discussing her X-rays, seems baffling. But then he almost certainly said to himself that her case was different from his because of her family history.

The generalized contempt which Lawrence could sometimes express for those who belonged to consumptive families, as he mistakenly thought A. E. Housman did, was no barrier to his being consistently caring and attentive to individual consumptives he knew (the bitter quarrel with Mansfield being a special case). He wrote to Gertie Cooper regularly, doing his best to cheer her up when by Christmas 1926 she was still confined to bed. The trouble is, he consoled her, that doctors in a sanatorium will not let you get up until your temperature is consistently just below normal but he admitted that, by those criteria, he himself would be in bed for ever. Still, he told his sister Ada, much better a sanatorium for Gertie at Christmas than the cemetery. He hoped for better news in 1927 but Gertie's diseased left lung refused to heal and, since the right was healthy, the doctors suggested to her, not a pneumothorax or a thoracoplasty, but the drastic step of removing the diseased parts (there may have been reasons why collapsing the lung was impossible). Lawrence was dismayed and for once in his life utterly incapable of offering clear advice as to whether Gertie should or should not go ahead with the operation. Normally he was a forthright and decisive person, only too willing to tell people what they should do; but in this instance he told Gertie that her situation worried him too much, that he could not make a decision on her behalf, and that she would have to make up her own mind. When he received details of the operation—six ribs and glands in the neck removed in addition to parts or the whole of a lung—he was horrified and wondered what, after so much damage to the body, there could be left. It goes without saying that Lawrence was a highly imaginative individual. Once when he was in Mexico he suddenly developed a wildly hysterical revulsion to staying in a certain town after reading that only a few years before the local employers had called a meeting of strikers, locked the building where the meeting was held, and then set fire to it. Reviewing a book on Pedro di Valdivia by R. B. Cunninghame Graham at the end of 1926, he implied that, in the descriptions of how Valdivia dealt with 'rebel' Indians in Peru, its author shared the insensitivity of the Spanish *conquistadores* without having their excuse. 'Imagine' he wrote, 'deliberately chopping off one slender brown Indian hand after another! Imagine taking a dark-haired Indian by the hair, cutting off his nose! Imagine seeing man after man, in the prime of life, with his mutilated face streaming blood, and his wrist stump a fountain of blood...'. These were episodes Lawrence clearly *could* imagine just as he imagined what Gertie Cooper must have gone through, from the accounts her friends sent him. He felt that for himself the cemetery *was* preferable, and that he would rather die. 'Why not chloroform and the long sleep!', he exclaimed to Koteliansky, 'Why save life in this ghastly way?'; and he told his older sister Emily, 'It's really better to die: if only one could die quickly.' Major surgery was not what he had expected when he had urged Gertie to have herself treated and arranged for her to go to the Mundesley. What happened to her was hardly likely to make him keener to take the same route especially as it was September 1927 before she was back with Ada in Ripley, a year after she had first left. Yet, although Gertie was born in 1885 and therefore Lawrence's exact contemporary, with her one healthy lung she managed to live twelve years longer than he did.

5

Alternative Medicine

When there is no effective and simple drug treatment for a disease (assuming drug treatment can ever be simple), and when the surgical options are dangerous or uncertain in outcome, the field is more than usually open for alternative medicine. The term is a loose one, difficult to define. The X-ray treatment Katherine Mansfield endured would now be regarded as a distinctly alternative option, and a very poor one at that; yet it was administered from at least the fringes of the medical establishment. The cowshed at the Gurdjieff Institute, on the other hand, lay definitely outside it. When Lawrence was obliged to give up the teaching profession at the beginning of 1912 because he was 'threatened with consumption', his colleagues presented him with a collection of Chekhov short stories. During his years as a tuberculosis patient Chekhov, himself a doctor, was prescribed arsenic, potassium bromide, koumiss, choral hydrate, guaiacol, Spanish fly, and camphor oil in very probable addition to the atropine, quinine, creosote, and ipecacuanha he had previously seen given to his dying, consumptive brother. Several of these substances must have been administered with the limited ambition of alleviating symptoms but some were regarded as steps forward towards a cure. In that capacity they would now be thought of as poor alternatives to bed rest because they were likely to have had no positive effects, and very possibly several adverse ones.

Although Lawrence ignored the 1925 diagnosis, or ignored its implications, he knew that he was ill and was very willing to take steps to get better, as long as they did not involve going into a sanatorium. He refused to believe what the Mexico City doctors told him yet took their advice about returning to the ranch rather than England, and from then on he was usually found in places thought at the time to be suitable for those suffering from tuberculosis, or (he might have added) from any severe chest complaint. After his six months at the ranch in New Mexico, he tried the effect of mountain air quite often. At the beginning of 1928, for example, the Lawrences joined Aldous and Julian Huxley, with their respective wives, at the skiing resort of Les Diablerets in Switzerland. Julian had by this time given up teaching zoology at London's King's College because H. G. Wells had been able to offer him a remarkable £10,000 for help in the preparation of a three-volumed handbook of biology, and his involvement in that project provided plenty of opportunities for those arguments about science which Aldous remembered in his preface to the 1932 edition of Lawrence's letters. Most of the rest of the time was devoted to winter sports in which Lawrence could not take part because of his condition, but he was nevertheless relatively contented and well in Les Diablerets. The experience encouraged him to take a chalet above the village of Gsteig, which is not far away, six months later; but there he was much less happy and when in the autumn of 1929 he spent some time in Rottach, in the Bavarian Alps, he was positively miserable. These differences can easily be attributed to his steadily worsening state but they are also a sign of how he increasingly felt the disadvantages of the mountain air alternative. The more emaciated he became the more he felt the cold. A once very active man, he relished exercise but now to move at all he needed to be on the flat and not in an area where steep inclines could quickly take away what little breath he had left.

After Mexico City, the next major crisis in Lawrence's health was the haemorrhage he suffered at the Villa Mirenda in July 1927. At the ranch in 1924 he is described by Dorothy Brett as spitting blood but this time it streamed from his mouth, as it had done from that of Katherine Mansfield just before she died. It was yet another of his very close calls and one he attributed, in writing to Gertler, to bronchial congestion. He claimed that the Florence doctor agreed with him in thinking that there was no need for sanatorium treatment but it is more likely that, with Gertie Cooper's example in mind, he heard, or persuaded the doctor to say, what he wanted to hear. The possibility of a sanatorium came up again three months later and was again rejected. This was when he was convalescing in Baden-Baden, where his mother-in-law lived, and took what was for him the major step of having himself examined by one of that town's many specialists. It was after this examination that he let slip that his lung had healed whereas previously he had never acknowledged there was anything wrong with it. Of the many treatments other than the sanatorium on offer for whatever had nearly killed him in July, and which still continued to make life uncertain and uncomfortable, he chose a short course of inhalations. From the very beginning of the fight against tuberculosis there had always been a great variety of these but at the particular establishment in Baden-Baden that

Lawrence briefly attended, the novelty lay in breathing in vapour from an underground spring known to contain radium. This proved no more beneficial for Lawrence than X-rays had for Mansfield. He felt better for a few days but then the effects wore off which is perhaps just as well given the damage inhaling radium can cause.

Sitting in a closed room with other sufferers in white robes and hoods, whom he could barely see through mists of vapour, was the nearest Lawrence would get to a sanatorium before the last month of his life; but although he refused that supposed way to recovery, he was not averse to regularly dosing himself with patent medicines. The time and cost they represented was after all minimal, and they might just work. His favourite among the hundreds of concoctions on the market was for a long time a French medicine known as *Solution Pantanberge*, an unsweetened mixture of creosote and chalk which was believed to harden tissue and fight off colds (he recommended it to Gertie Cooper). In 1928, on Gertie's counter recommendation, his sister sent him some Umckaloaba which he obediently took without feeling it did him much good ('Perhaps it doesn't go for one's bronchials'). This was a famous or at least notorious medicine, the subject in England of court cases and parliamentary enquiry. It had been developed by a Major C. H. Stevens and its purpose was evident from his having formed a 'Consumption Cure' company. Scores of tuberculosis sufferers testified that it had restored them to perfect health, even though the scientists from the British Medical Association who analysed the product could find nothing of value in it. The loud and often violent public debates about the therapeutic virtues of Umckaloaba helped to make it an exceptionally profitable venture, and also inspired H. G. Well's *Tono-Bungay*. This lively novel appeared in 1909 and tells the story of a provincial chemist who becomes very rich by marketing bottles of a tonic which the narrator describes as 'slightly injurious rubbish', the 'Tono-Bungay' of the title. As a young man Lawrence was very keen on early Wells and especially *Tono-Bungay*. He called it a great book which friends should use to form their judgement of Wells rather than the 'arrant rot' of his science fiction. But as he dissolved in water the capsules his sister had sent him and drank the results, he does not seem to have recalled what the novel was about, or made the connection with what he was drinking.

Lawrence may have been tempted to accord more credence to Umckaloaba than its effect on him suggested it deserved because he had heard about its origins. Identified as a prospective consumptive himself, Major Stevens had been sent to South Africa where a black African healer had cured him with a mysterious drink made from boiled roots. Umckaloaba, he learned, was the African name for this drink and he would not later have found it strange that its properties should escape the attention of such an obvious representative of Western science as a BMA analyst. A man like Wells was that analyst's natural ally and felt that, if people could only demonstrate a sufficient degree of political intelligence and will, the progress of science and technology must eventually lead to an increasingly comfortable and therefore happy existence for mankind. But Lawrence had little faith in a Wellsian vision of the future and believed that the past was not just a stepping stone to a better life but a repository of lost truths. Even when he first went to Italy with Frieda, before she was divorced from her first husband Ernest Weekley, he felt that he had found in the small villages where they lived a traditional way of life with values and understandings fast disappearing from an increasingly industrialized Britain. The First World War shattered whatever belief he might have retained in progress, scientific or otherwise. After it was over, and he was living in New Mexico, he was at first suspicious of the Indians who preserved to an astonishing degree non-Western habits and rituals in their pueblos around Taos; but he gradually came to appreciate and admire what these stood for. More generally, he became convinced that before Socrates and Jesus, the two figures who he regarded as the founders of Western culture, there had been a now lost science more in tune with the real needs and aspirations of human beings than its contemporary version. With attitudes like these it is hardly surprising that, when it came to questions of health and medicine, Lawrence should have displayed a marked preference for folk remedies of the kind he remembered his father taking. When he came back to the Villa Mirenda from Baden-Baden in 1927 he brought with him a *Brust-thee*, a herbal tea for chest conditions (Germany was, as it still is, a great centre for herbal remedies). Following the instructions, he would boil up this tea slowly for the prescribed number of hours and was as faithful to it as he had been to *Solution Pantanberge*.

Lawrence's preference for folk medicine over its official version can only have been strengthened by the story of Frieda's ankle. It was in April 1929, while he was briefly testing out the Majorca where ninety years before George Sand had nursed an increasingly tubercular Chopin, that the ankle was badly sprained; and Frieda was still limping when in June she went to London for the opening of an exhibition of Lawrence's paintings. He himself was too unwell for such a long journey and also apprehensive that recent troubles over *Lady Chatterley's Lover,* and other of his writings, might lead to his being arrested. Frieda was treated in London by a Harley Street specialist and then later, because there was no improvement, by a doctor in Baden-Baden. When she and Lawrence were in Rottach in the autumn, he was both delighted and enraged to see the village 'bone-setter' give his wife's ankle a firm knock back into place. The delight came from the fact that Frieda immediately began to improve and was soon as good as new. The rage was a consequence both of the bone-setter saying that, had he not acted when he did, Frieda would have limped for the rest of her life, and of the Harley Street specialist having charged 12 guineas (with the bill from Baden-Baden still outstanding).

Lawrence went to Rottach in order to see a German admirer called Max Mohr, who was himself a doctor as well as a writer. It is an indication of how unwell he felt there that he allowed his well-connected sister-in-law to send three more doctors from Munich to see him. Frieda had two sisters. Johanna, the younger, was a socialite who had first married an army officer and then a banker; but the elder, Else, had a Ph.D. from Heidelberg and moved in both academic and political circles (her husband had been a professor of economics who was very briefly the Bavarian finance minister at the end of the First World War). She knew scores of artists and scientists and it had no doubt been because of her that, in the autumn of 1927 when he was staying in a holiday house near Munich which she owned, he had been visited by Hans Carossa, a prominent writer as well as a doctor with a special interest in tuberculosis. Lawrence reported that Carossa's stethoscope could pick up nothing from the lungs, which they both concluded must therefore have healed, so that 'there was only the bronchials—and doctors aren't a bit interested in bronchials'. Yet a writer friend who had accompanied Carossa on this 1927 visit claimed later to have asked him what the real situation was, and been told, 'An average man with those lungs would have died long ago. But with a real artist no normal prognosis is really sure. There are other forces involved. Maybe Lawrence can live two or three years more. But no medical treatment can really save him.'

Of the three doctors who were sent to see him two years later in Rottach, Lawrence chose to rely on the least orthodox. He had been a priest and claimed he would be able to cure Lawrence completely through a combination of diet and breathing exercises. His body, this doctor claimed, had been poisoned with unsuitable food and it was the effect of this food on the vagus nerve which caused the constant breathlessness. He prescribed porridges of millet, barley, or oatmeal with lots of fresh fruit and vegetables; roast beef but no coffee, vinegar, pastries, or rich sauces. In addition he said that his patient should take small doses of arsenic and phosphorus twice a day. After a week of doing this, Lawrence gave up the doses on the reasonable grounds that this time he felt he really *was* being poisoned. He persisted with the diet much longer but with decreasing optimism. Three weeks after leaving Rottach for Bandol, he complained of the ground he felt he had lost in Germany and said he would never go north again. 'And the doctors,' he added, 'they can do nothing for one. They are merely a fraud.'

What may have initially encouraged Lawrence to try the diet treatment which the priest-doctor offered was that he had often had trouble with his digestive system. When he was gravely ill during his trip to Sri Lanka to see the Brewsters in 1923, he said that in all his thirty-six years his insides had never hurt him so much and the context makes clear that he was referring to his bowels. When he fell dangerously ill in Oaxaca in 1925, he described himself as having been shot in the intestines. His complaints on both occasions may have been unconnected with tuberculosis but later digestive troubles could well have been a result of his disease having spread downwards from his lungs. In the common use of the word tuberculosis 'pulmonary' is generally understood, but most parts of the body are of course vulnerable to its attack. Kafka had his first tubercular haemorrhage in 1917 and from then on spent a good deal of his time in sanatoria: far from being accused of denial, it has been claimed that he gave an obscure welcome to his illness because it allowed him to escape his engagement to Felice Bauer and satisfied his sense of his own unworthiness. Matters progressed as at that period they usually did but in 1924 there was a dramatic worsening of his condition when the tuberculosis spread upwards from the lungs to his larynx. This prevented him from eating and he was dead within two months, partly from starvation. The more common direction of the disease was downwards and a consequence of the ingestion of infected sputum. Andrew Morland reported in 1932 that in post-mortems on patients who had died from pulmonary tuberculosis over 50 per cent were found to have the disease in their intestines also. This was a condition Chekhov was able to diagnose in himself and when he followed a treatment of four bottles a day of koumiss (fermented mare's milk), it was not only because it allowed him to gain twelve pounds but also that it encouraged the growth of benign flora at the expense of the tuberculosis bacilli in the gut. The benefits were short-lived and his last months were made unbearable not only by constant coughing but also by diarrhoea. Lawrence is reticent about his digestive or bowel troubles but there is no doubt that he found it difficult to eat properly, even though he was alarmed by his continual loss of weight. The idea that he had been trying to eat the wrong foods, and it was this effort rather than the body which received them that was at fault, might therefore have had a special appeal for him.

It was an appeal which did not last and one more failed alternative for a man fast running out of them. But then this was because he had set himself some limits. In Shakespeare's *All's Well That Ends Well*, the King of France has consulted all the best doctors as only kings can and is so convinced he is dying that, when a young doctor's daughter arrives with her offer of a miracle cure, his first impulse is to send her away. He says that he does not want to 'prostitute' his 'past-cure malady to empirics', or to so dissever 'our great self and our credit, to esteem | A senseless help when help past sense we deem.' The lines have an awkwardness characteristic of this play but also a jagged force powerful enough to bring to mind the intolerable dilemma of someone in the last stages of a fatal illness who is trapped between 'What harm could it do?', on the one hand, and 'Have I not the courage to face up to the truth?', on the other hand. Lawrence listened when a friend of Murry's whom Dorothy Brett had insisted he meet extolled the virtues of Gurdjieff, and he made a point of visiting the Fontainebleau Institute when he was staying in Paris in 1924. But he then decided that Gurdjieff was a crank who could do nothing for him. During his stay in Baden-Baden in 1928, Frieda spoke of a nun from a local convent who effected miraculous cures by the laying on of hands. He might then have done what many have done in a similar situation and said, 'Well, if *you* insist . . . '; but instead he dismissed outright the possibility of seeing the nun. Lawrence would not have called his own self 'great' in quite the way Shakespeare's king does, but for him also, there were alternatives incompatible with his ability to maintain his respect for it.

6

Being Ill

Whatever he tried, Lawrence's health continued to deteriorate. As time went by, his periods of remission became shorter and shorter. And yet, as he must often have reminded himself, it was only in September 1925 that he had turned 40. He needed some explanation for his situation apart from the obvious one adopted by many of his friends that he was dying. What he was experiencing, he often insisted, was the male menopause: a period of biological change and disruption which was essentially transitional, the difficult pathway to a calmer time. One of the reasons that the optimistic claims of the diet doctor from Munich temporarily triumphed over Lawrence's strong natural scepticism was that he told his patient that most men between the ages of 42 and 49 had to endure great changes in their 'animal man'. This is what Lawrence firmly believed even though the signs of changes in him were so much more dramatic than in his friends of a similar age. Aldous Huxley could tell him that there was nothing in the biological textbooks about a male menopause but Lawrence was older than Huxley by nearly ten years and felt he was in a position to know better.

The male menopause was an organic explanation for his illness but Lawrence had no difficulty in combining or reinforcing it with his long-standing belief that people fell ill because they did not know how to live. 'One is ill', he had had Birkin say in *Women in Love,* 'because one doesn't live properly—can't. It's the failure to live that makes one ill, and humiliates one.' In the middle 1920s, failing to live properly increasingly came to mean having been too concerned to change other people and reform the world. This is what Frieda would scathingly refer to as Lawrence's *salvator mundi* touch. He deals with it directly in the first part of *The Man Who Died,* a novella originally entitled *The Escaped Cock.* Though the context is naturalistic ('They took me down too soon,' explains the Jesus figure), this is a retelling of the resurrection story and allows Lawrence to describe vividly what it feels like to come back from the brink of extinction, as he had so often done himself. Once restored to health, the man of the story decides that he has in the past been far too concerned with proselytizing, and that he ought now to make the most of the phenomenal world and live free of care, something Lawrence himself often said he wanted to do after 1925. He became convinced that his mother's cancer had been brought on not only by repression of the natural feelings but also by anxiety, stress, or worry, by caring too much. As he pondered the reasons for his own ill health, to be more carefree and insouciant became one of his own chief aims. The power of the mind could thus be demonstrated in not only defying disease, or denying it was really there, but also in altering the conditions which brought it about.

Yet it was not easy for Lawrence to give up caring. Like Birkin, he often seemed doomed to what is described in *Women in Love* as the 'old effort at serious living'. During the early 1920s he had been intensely preoccupied with what kind of political organization could best help to heal the wounds of the post-war world, and in novels like *Kangaroo* or *The Plumed Serpent* he both explored and advocated blueprints of his own. It was just after he had finished his second and final version of *The Plumed Serpent* in Oaxaca that he collapsed and from then on his interest in changing the world through political action waned, as did his interest in novel-writing generally. He had cared too much and, give or take a few enthusiastic young disciples, the only result was that he was now unwell. When in October 1926 he began writing about a gamekeeper and the young wife of a crippled English aristocrat, what he had in mind was a novella. But by the time he was busy with a third version of this story more than a year later, it had become a novel and one which was unpublishable in any usual fashion because of explicit descriptions of sexual intercourse and the liberal use of words like cunt and fuck. After arranging to have the novel published privately in Florence, Lawrence threw himself energetically into the task of sending copies to subscribers in Britain, the United States, and elsewhere. When the inevitable denunciations came, and he was accused of being a pornographer, making sure that as many people as possible had access to *Lady Chatterley's Lover*, and defending it against its enemies, was a task he pursued with missionary zeal. From having been deeply concerned about the political future of the world, he became fervently preoccupied with showing through both his novel and what he said in defence of it, that more openness about sex was an essential condition for a better life. However much he may have wanted or intended to relax, here was a new subject which kept him just as active, involved, and concerned as he had previously tended to be. In her biography of Lawrence, Catherine Carswell describes how on one occasion he wrote to her and said that he did not 'give a damn for any blooming thing'. The kind of mood these words suggest, she shrewdly notes, was with him usually a preliminary 'to caring ardently for some one thing in particular'.

Lawrence had always had trouble with censorship. In his early years he seems often to have stumbled into difficulty, writing the truth as he saw it and only later realizing that it caused offence in certain quarters. There was by contrast a degree of challenge and provocation in the way he composed *Lady Chatterley's Lover* (the same kind of spirit which led him to say that he always put a phallus somewhere in his paintings in order to shock 'people's castrated social spirituality'). He was able to post the novel to customers in Britain before the authorities quite knew what was happening; but they then retaliated by seizing a package of his which contained a volume in typescript of relatively innocuous poems. When he showed his paintings in London, they closed the exhibition down on the pretext that many of his nudes were depicted with pubic hair. By that time Lawrence was in open warfare with the British moral establishment and becoming inured to all the unpleasant things said about him in the popular press. As a young man he had suffered agonies of self-consciousness at the thought of how exposed any one of his writings left him; but over time he had grown used to being talked about in public, even when the talk was unfriendly. Some insults hurt nevertheless. Shortly before their first stay in Bandol, the Lawrences had accepted an invitation from their friend Richard Aldington to spend some time on Port Cros, a small island opposite the town of Hyères (which is also on the French Mediterranean coast). The visit was not a success and had to be curtailed, in part because Aldington had borrowed a property which was on the top of a hill and there was a forty-five-minute trek down to the beach. This was simple enough for the others there, but impossible for Lawrence who therefore found himself as immobilized as he had been in the mountains of Switzerland or Germany. One evening the whole company gathered round the fire while Lawrence looked over some of the reviews of *Lady Chatterley's Lover* which had been sent to him from England. After pondering them for some time he muttered to himself, 'Nobody *likes* being called a cesspool', and he then began manically piling wood on the fire until he was in danger of burning the house down.

Telling a friend in April 1929 that he was going to Majorca because his cough was no better, Lawrence remarked 'Jix would say it's my sins—I say it's his' ('Jix' being the nickname of Sir William Joynson-Hicks, the British Home Secretary who oversaw questions of censorship). This was a third way Lawrence had of explaining why his health refused to improve. He was ill because he was experiencing the male menopause and because in the past he had caused himself stress by caring too much. But he was also ill because of the persecutions he had been obliged to endure, persecutions which were among the simpler of those 'wounds to the soul' he refers to in his poem 'Healing'. And yet although Lawrence remained sensitive to insult and injury, he was also a naturally combative person who relished a fight and of whom it could therefore be said that his enemies kept him alive. 'Just as with the ancient Cynics', Nietzsche wrote of Schopenhauer, 'his rage was his balm, his recreation, his compensation, his specific against tedium, in short, his happiness.' In Huxley's view, rage was for Lawrence a specific not so much against tedium as against the 'secret consciousness of his dissolution' which otherwise filled 'the

last years of his life with an overpowering sadness'. Enemies like Jix
were therefore useful in keeping that rage at an appropriate level.
This is a psychological view of the role which rage or anger played in
Lawrence's illness but David Garnett, who had trained as a biologist,
had a more organic one. Talking in old age about the fits of anger
which he had often seen Lawrence display, he said that they were
useful because they stimulated an extra flow of adrenalin which was
known to keep the tubercular bacillus at bay. Any tuberculosis
sufferer overhearing this dubious claim would have had a right to
feel confused. The doctors told you to go to the mountains and to
some warm spot on the Mediterranean coast; they said you should
above all rest and avoid stress but also (if they were like Garnett) that
you could prolong your life by losing your temper.

Lawrence wanted to stay alive in order to fight his enemies but
also to defeat their expectations. The frequency with which he
insisted that there was nothing wrong with his lungs suggests he
knew that other people thought of him as a consumptive and, as
his own remarks on Housman indicate, he was familiar with what
was expected of such people. In both the official and popular mind
tuberculosis was associated with sexual licence. 'Sexual vice is one
horror', said a council member for the National Association for the
Prevention of Tuberculosis in 1912, 'the alcoholic habit another,
and the two are seldom found apart from the tubercle.' *The Magic
Mountain* suggests that the idea of some close association between
sexuality and tuberculosis was at least encouraged, if not initiated,
by large numbers of young people, who were only intermittently
ill, being shut up in sanatoria where there was often very little to
do; but Mann also hints that there might, in his view, be some link
between heightened sexual activity and the fevers that tuberculosis

patients habitually ran. The danger for Lawrence was that *Lady Chatterley's Lover* would be regarded as a typical expression of a consumptive rather than the brave statement of sexual openness he wanted it to be. 'Lawrence was not', said Curtis Brown, the head of his literary agency, 'an erotomaniac. In various delightful talks with him on all sorts of subjects, *that* subject never once presented itself. But it is likely that his tuberculosis, with its well known bearing on sex impulses, may have led his eye unusually often to that subject, and once focussed on it, we had *Lady Chatterley's Lover.*' Lawrence would have been well aware of attitudes like this, even in educated people like Curtis Brown. The best way to defeat them was first to insist that he did not have tuberculosis, or at least in any form which was life-threatening; and then to make sure that he stayed alive. There is a story that Voltaire once refused to go out in a thunderstorm and, when accused of cowardice, said that he did not want to risk being struck by lightning because dying in that way would give too much satisfaction to the priests who were his enemies. Lawrence had analogous reasons for not wanting to die of tuberculosis. No one likes to be stereotyped or to hear murmuring in the background the smug superiority of 'I told you so'.

It was not only from the direction of his enemies that he could hear variations of this murmur. After the episode in Paris when Lawrence had broken the appointment to have an X-ray, the Huxleys were gravely perturbed. The next time they were in England, they must have often said how worried they were. The result was a batch of letters from England in which friends expressed concern, offered advice, and generally made clear their assumption that he must be in a very bad way. Lawrence was forced to write back and say he was not dead yet, but later he complained to Orioli, 'How they do like to dwell on the thought of my being dead.' He said they had all determined he should die 'so of course I shall live a hundred years, and put wreaths on their graves'. It was bad enough when friends made clear they did not expect him to survive but worse to remember that this expectation had once come from closer home. In one of several short descriptions of his family background written in the last years of his life, Lawrence recalled that after the publication of his first novel (*The White Peacock*), a London editor had written to his mother and told her that her son would be riding in his own carriage by the time he was 40. 'Ay', he had heard his mother had said, 'if he lives to forty.' Writing in 1926, Lawrence went on to point out that he had managed to do that—which was 'one in the eye for that sighing remark'—and that, although his health had always been weak, what he called his 'life' remained strong. 'Why had they all made up their minds that I was to die?' he asked himself, and he replied, 'Perhaps they thought I was too good to live. Well, in that case they were had!' His angry determination was that his present friends and enemies should be had also.

Lawrence was made angry by the hostilities he encountered, and by the nature of the categories into which he felt others placed him; but there is another variety of anger which comes from being sick when others around you remain healthy: from the injustice of falling ill when people who are of the same age, or older, are able to press on regardless. This is the feeling memorably captured in Tolstoy's *The Death of Ivan Ilyich*, but it is also central to the story Somerset Maugham wrote about his stay in the sanatorium near Aberdeen in 1919. In that, one of the fellow patients of

Ashenden—Maugham's narrator and alter ego—is a stocky, broad-shouldered accountant in his mid-thirties who is happily married with two children, has worked in the City, lived a regular life, and seemed the unlikeliest of candidates for tuberculosis. His devoted wife visits him every week but he treats her more and more cruelly and eventually tells her not to come because, as he explains to Ashenden, he cannot bear to see her so 'strong and well and full of beans'. It takes the example of a fellow patient, in the terminal phases of his disease, but determined to live as fully as he can, to persuade the accountant to accept the unfairness of his situation and change his attitude. In Philip Roth's 2006 novel *Everyman*, the protagonist has been devoted to his elder brother but finds that, as his own health deteriorates, he can no longer speak to him because he so angrily resents his brother's continuing vitality and well-being.

Whatever feelings of this kind Lawrence might have experienced, they are very rarely expressed, yet there is one occasion when they do surface, although in a much less unreasonable form than those of Maugham's accountant or Roth's hero. Lawrence had always had good relations with older women and he got on particularly well with his mother-in-law. Their beginnings had not been auspicious. The Baroness von Richthofen was hardly delighted when her daughter left the respectable, middle-class Englishman by whom she had had three children and turned up in Germany with a writer who was almost six years her junior, of uncertain health, and even more uncertain prospects. But things turned out better than expected and the Baroness warmed to Lawrence as time went by. While never attaining the fluency of Frieda's first husband, who was after all a professor of modern languages, he mastered enough German to write her long gossipy letters, contrived to send money during the difficult period of hyper-inflation after the war when the savings of most Germans were swept away, and was always attentive to her needs. It was not mere duty which prompted him in these attentions but an enjoyment of her company which lasted until their final meeting. This was in July 1929, in Baden-Baden, when the Baroness was looking forward to spending some time in a spa hotel in the mountains about an hour's journey away. Lawrence by this time was too ill to want to move and had in any case lost most of his faith in mountains, but his mother-in-law pressurized him and Frieda into taking her to them. He gives a grotesquely vivid picture of how the old lady, once she was at the spa, stood in the roadway gulping in cold mountain air and exclaiming, 'Es gibt mir Kraft, es gibt mir Kraft' (It gives me strength). Her behaviour seemed to him to indicate an insane selfishness born of a hideous terror of having to die and he angrily resented the fact that the strength the Baroness was seeking might well be at his expense (having to leave the comfortable hotel in Baden-Baden had worsened his state). He told a friend that he knew his mother-in-law would secretly gloat if he died at 43 and she managed to live on at 78—that she would then feel an ugly triumph. It must have struck him as especially unjust that, whereas someone almost twice his age could comfortably gulp down air in great mouthfuls, he often had to fight hard for every breath. He felt angry at the measures she was taking to survive him, as in fact she did. Like Lawrence, the Baroness also died in 1930 but in November, outliving him by several months.

7

Death and the After-Life

L awrence refused to regard his illness as terminal yet in the late 1920s death was a subject which increasingly preoccupied him. His attitude to it was very different from his mother's. One of the reasons he felt able to deny or neglect his tuberculosis may have been the consciousness of coming from a family it had never directly affected. It was in her late fifties that his mother died of cancer but his father was an unusually healthy and vigorous man who began working in the pit at the age of 10 and was still there more than fifty years later (he died when he was 77). Both his sisters were healthy and so was his oldest sibling, George. There had been only one early death in the family, that of his brother Ernest who at the time was its undoubted star. An athlete, Ernest had done very well at school and at the age of 22 was living in London and launched on what looked like being a successful business career. But he then fell ill from some unknown cause, the most startling symptom of which was the skin disorder known as erysipelas, and died so quickly that tuberculosis could be ruled out (characteristically Lawrence would later claim that the real cause was worry and psychological conflict). The devastating effect of Ernest's death on his mother, who idolized him, and who may also have been relying on him to fulfil her dreams of social advancement, is dramatized in *Sons and Lovers*. Mrs Lawrence later confided to the mother of Jessie Chambers that she looked forward to meeting Ernest in Heaven more than Jesus Christ himself.

In our time, a remark like this can only sound quaint, but the belief that death would mean a reunion with lost loved ones has been remarkably widespread in the past and was held by many with minds far more sophisticated than Mrs Lawrence's. As Pascal approached death, for example, he looked forward to meeting again his father, his sister Jacqueline, and the mother whom he had known too little. The comfort that such an expectation provided is incalculable but whatever the degree, it must have considerably lessened the terrors of dying. To be deprived of it was a major change in the human condition. The difference is not solely due to there being fewer Christians than there were but to the fact that Christianity and the notion of immortality are not now so closely linked. Questioned on the topic of life after death, for example, the Archbishop of Canterbury has recently said that it is not 'a function of something in us that survives but something to do with our doctrine of God'. He nevertheless went on to add that what Christians call the resurrection of the body involves God 'giving another shape, another carrier, another vehicle, to the information complex that is the life we have lived', but what that shape was, and how continuity was maintained between this life and the next, was a question on which 'we haven't a clue'. The more, he concluded, life after death was about the character of God rather than our potentially dual nature, the less vulnerable it was to 'straight scientific criticism'. That may well be true but making it less vulnerable, and talking of the body as an information complex, considerably lessens the succour Christian doctrine can bring to those who grieve, or who are about to die.

The effect of Lawrence's own religious upbringing is apparent in the biblical rhythms of his prose, his familiarity with the Bible stories, and his fondness for hymns or songs associated with the Church like the Temperance favourite 'Throw out the life-line | Some-one is sinking today'. A gifted mimic, he would in later life sing these words while throwing out an imaginary life-line to drowning souls, and then pretend to haul them in strenuously. His mother would have been appalled and felt that he was the one who was drowning. Lawrence lost his Christian faith in his early twenties but was never entirely comfortable without it. In *The Rainbow* Ursula Brangwen echoes his own position when she cannot believe the college physics teacher who tells her that life consists in a complex of physical and chemical activities to which there is no need to attribute any special mystery. Lawrence felt that many Christian doctrines were fatally undermined by the science of his day, and he found no way of reconciling the idea of a benevolent deity with the indiscriminate allocation of suffering in the world; but rejecting the dogmas of the Church was easier than ridding himself of a religious temperament and the belief that there were powers in the universe not indifferent to human life. The dilemma was a familiar one in his time and helps to explain the appeal of Gurdjieff, or other purveyors of substitute faiths such as the enormously successful Madame Blavatsky, founder of a mish-mash of Eastern and Western religions known as Theosophy.

Lawrence was very interested in Theosophy, as in several other similar movements, but unlike W. B. Yeats he was never formally enrolled. He would have said with William Blake that he needed to create his own system in order not to be enslaved by someone else's. His chief complaint was that Theosophy was too mystical, not sufficiently down to earth; and yet in an introduction he wrote for his *Fantasia of the Unconscious* in 1922 he found himself driven to confess a position which was not very down to earth either. 'I am sorry to say', he then wrote, 'I believe in the souls of the dead. I am almost ashamed to say I believe the souls of the dead in some way re-enter life and pervade the souls of the living.' What seems to have motivated this shamefaced avowal is that, in the years following her death, Lawrence (a vivid dreamer) was quite literally haunted by his mother. She and other people he had known appeared to him so frequently in his dreams that he found it impossible to dismiss their apparition as a merely psychological phenomenon: an extension of the classical humanist position (to which he also subscribed) that if we live on after our deaths it is only in the minds of other people. To the end of his life he remained interested in ghosts and wrote several stories in which they figure; and yet at a time when the Spiritualist movement had been reinvigorated by the adherence of Arthur Conan Doyle, and the loss of so many lives during the First World War, he showed no more interest in joining it than he had in becoming a Theosophist.

Lawrence may have believed in the spirits of the dead yet it is hard to find any clear sign in his life or writing of a firm conviction that his own spirit would live on. One of the few works of philosophy we can be certain he read was a selection of Schopenhauer's essays translated by Mrs Rudolf Dircks. He and Jessie Chambers pored over this pocket-sized volume and must have noticed the 'Short dialogue on the indestructibility of true being by death'. One of the speakers in this piece argues that we are all immortal because the matter of which we are composed is absorbed back into the world at our death to be made use of again. It is very much in terms of this argument that Lawrence wrote to his sister Ada in 1911 when she also was beginning to lose her faith. He told her that when she died she would be like a raindrop falling back into the sea, 'the big shimmering sea of unorganised life which we call God'; and that, though we are then lost as individuals, we 'count in the whole'.

An advantage of this familiar view is that it is consistent with the scientific principle of the indestructibility of matter but many of its critics have pointed out that, once we accept the first part of the proposition (being lost as individuals), it is hard to have much interest in the second. If we are lost in that way how can we be said to count at all? Lawrence was, however, able to give the position a more optimistic turn as, during the 1920s, his views became increasingly animistic. What impressed him about the American Indians he observed in New Mexico was the way they were able to avoid the fatal matter/spirit, body/soul dualism of Western culture by treating their gods as not 'in' or 'behind' the natural world but identical with it. This meant that death was also for them a return to God in the Schopenhauerean sense yet, as their rituals emphasized, although such a return might well be permanent, it could also be part of a natural cycle of birth, death, and renewal, the cycle of the seasons. One might be merged and lost forever or only temporarily lost until the next spring. Thinking of his own case in these terms was consistent with regarding his illness as no more than an uncomfortable transitional phase. It is not hard to detect Lawrence doing this in many of the texts he wrote in the last years of his life. In the second half of *The Man Who Died*, for example, the Jesus figure is nursed back into full life by a priestess of Isis with whom he has a brief sexual experience. In the form of the story Lawrence favoured, Isis is the brother of Osiris, the parts of whose body have been widely scattered. Every year it is her task to gather these parts together because once she has found them, the genitalia last of all, the Nile will flood and prosperity will return to the land. This is a fertility myth from Egypt which captured his imagination but in his beautiful poem *Bavarian Gentians* he turns to the Greek story of Persephone, dragged down to the underworld by Hades during the winter but allowed to return to earth in spring. When he is exploring how periods of darkness and apparent extinction can be followed by light, just as winter is eventually followed by brighter days, or whether living as closely in tune with the rhythms of Nature as possible might allow one to participate in her resilience, everything is grist to his mill. In matters of religious belief he is nothing if not eclectic.

Lawrence's favourite symbol of renewal was the mythological phoenix, able to consume itself in fire yet rise again from the ashes. More directly observable was the almond tree. Behind the villa in which he and Frieda had lived in Taormina was a grove of almond trees which has now been replaced by unattractive buildings (its present owner remembers how when he was a boy he was paid by his uncle to knock down the nuts with a stick). Lawrence found the sight of these trees in winter particularly unpromising and described their branches in a poem as like 'bare iron hooks'. In January or February therefore it delighted him to see that 'even iron can put forth . . . puff with clouds of blossom'. What this phenomenon must have suggested to him was that cases which seem hopeless might not necessarily be so. There were plenty of almond trees in the Bandol area also, including those in the garden of the villa which his friends the Brewsters eventually succeeded in renting, but at the beginning of 1930 he was too ill to go out to see them as they began to puff their clouds of blossom. He must then have been apprehensive that he would be excluded from the annual miracle of renewal.

And yet how could a man like Lawrence ever die when his mind still teemed with thoughts and images? Writers characteristically live in a world of imagined landscapes, encounters, and scenarios even—if he is anything to go by—when they are asleep ('I am a devil at dreaming,' he once said). They are by definition people of super-active consciousness and therefore more likely than most to encounter the perils of solipsism. Lawrence was well aware of his own solipsistic tendencies and fought against them. In a poem called 'New Heaven and Earth', written during the war, he expresses very powerfully the nausea he felt in being trapped in a world of his own imaginings where everything was, as he puts it, 'tainted' with himself. What has saved him from this situation, he says, is touching the side of his wife in bed and realizing that there was something in the world which was not himself, that 'verily... was not me'. In a more decorous or puritanical age it was a wall or tree which Wordsworth remembered having to grab hold of as a child in order to save himself from solipsism, or what he describes, in an autobiographical note to the Immortality Ode, as an 'abyss of idealism'. But for Lawrence it was the body of a woman.

The more solipsistic the temperament, the more difficult it is for people to imagine they could ever die. 'I should have smiled pityingly', says Proust's narrator, 'had a philosopher expressed the idea that some day, even some distant day, I should have had to die; that the external forces of nature would survive me … that after me there would remain those rounded swelling cliffs, that sea, that moonlight and that sky; how was that possible; how could the world last longer than myself, since it was the world that was enclosed in me?' People who feel like this, Schopenhauer once commented, find it difficult to think of themselves as 'absolutely perishable in contrast to imperishable nature'. Yet 'New Heaven and Earth' shows that Lawrence was alive to the dangers of his own temperament and he had enough commonsense, as well as enough humour, to have appreciated the witty parody of the death-defying solipsist which the Housman whose 'Shropshire Lad' he had so deprecated published in 1936, too late for him to read:

> Good creatures, do you love your lives?
> and have you ears for sense?
> Here is a knife like other knives,
> that cost me eighteenpence.
> I need but stick it in my heart
> and down will come the sky.
> And earth's foundations will depart
> *and all you folk will die.*

If Lawrence was not to be saved by his solipsism, since even solipsists die, or by the miracle of annual renewal (any potential failure of which in his own case he could never *quite* believe), what did he imagine awaited him after death? In an effort to cheer him up, Frieda said at some point during the last weeks that they would both live to see jolly times once again, but Lawrence only replied that this would be 'in Heaven, my dear'. He did not in fact believe in Heaven, or any of the other features of Christian eschatology, but then neither could he quite accept the materialist view that after death the body decays and there is nothing more to be said. The precise details of his alternative position are, however, very hard to clarify, especially as what Blake would have called his 'system' can only be glimpsed through his creative writing and the odd casual remark. That the disparate items which compose it are taken from such a wide range of religions or mythologies is also perhaps not an aid to clarity.

Something of the problem can be seen in one of his best-known poems 'The Ship of Death', that mournful meditation on approaching dissolution which he composed shortly before he died. Reading any poem as an expression of an author's views is always hazardous but in this case the hazard is increased by the existence of several differing versions. The two principal ones both begin with references to autumn as the season of decay and death, with (as Lawrence memorably puts it) 'the bruised body, the frightened soul . . . shrinking, wincing from the cold | that blows upon it through the orifices'. He then introduces the ship of death itself, the boat from Egyptian mythology which has to contain provisions for a long voyage because it ferries dead souls to the after-life just as in Greek mythology those same souls are rowed across the Styx to the underworld by Charon (a figure of whom there are distinct echoes in at least one of the poem's versions). The destination of the souls is what Lawrence calls several times the sea of 'oblivion'. This is nearly always a very positive word for him. In earlier times he had yearned for oblivion as a welcome release from his relentless solipsism and in 'The Ship of Death' it is equated with what in one of the versions is described as 'utter peace'. It could be said that this definition represents a calm acceptance of future extinction, of death as the final elimination of all future hopes and fears; but it seems more likely that Lawrence regards oblivion as a state analogous to sleep whereas, as has often been pointed out, a chief characteristic of death in the sense of non-existence is that it is the end, the negation of all states. In any case Lawrence's oblivion does not mark the end of 'The Ship of Death'. In one version there is a dawn, 'the cruel dawn of coming back to life'; in another, after the 'lovely last, last lapse of death, into pure oblivion', only a question: 'But can it be that also it is procreation?' Since in the first of these instances, the poem goes on to speak of the body emerging 'strange and lovely' as the flood subsides, 'like a worn sea-shell', both these conditions which succeed oblivion could be regarded as familiar allusions in Lawrence to the hope of eventually recovering his health. But in a context where the prospect of a real rather than merely symbolic death seems so insistent, they could also be regarded as hints of some kind of after-life. Quite what the nature of that after-life would be is a topic on which Lawrence is no clearer than the present Archbishop of Canterbury, although his use of the English language is more appealing. In one of the versions of 'The Ship of Death' there are extended references to dissatisfied, unexpiated souls roaming 'like outcast dogs on the margins of life' and still able to trouble the living. This suggests a belief in the supernatural very like the one to which Lawrence directly confessed in *Fantasia of the Unconscious*. Yet the soul which has prepared properly for death can ignore these unfortunates and make the journey to the 'core of sheer oblivion' after which there is, on one reading, a new healthy body or, on another, a form of after-life which is beyond the power of humans to imagine. Definite about most subjects, everything Lawrence wrote suggests that, on the prospect of his own life after death, the right word to describe him is agnostic. All he knew, or at least felt, was that religion, in the widest sense of that word, had more to say about the questions which mattered most to him than modern science.

8

Ending it All

At the beginning of *The Rack*, the central character is understood by others to have congratulated himself on suffering from a disease which was at least painless but is told to reserve judgement until he has seen someone dying from tuberculosis. It was the nights which Lawrence found particularly hard to bear. After his first stay in Bandol, while Frieda went to Germany, he travelled up to Paris with a young Welsh admirer called Rhys Davies. A stop in a hotel on the way made Davies feel that he had never seen such a frail, wasted, and vulnerable-looking body as Lawrence's. Once in Paris he was woken by the sound of Lawrence's coughing in the next room and, when he went to help, found him 'as though in mortal combat with some terrible invisible opponent who had arrived in those mysterious dead hours that follow midnight'. His suggestion that he should call a doctor was vehemently refused but Lawrence asked Davies to sit with him a little and soon he was calmer and lay back exhausted: 'The opponent had gone.' This idea of disease as a battle with some alien occupying force was often Lawrence's own. In October 1929 he told Mabel Luhan how strongly he felt that his illness was not really him, 'yet there is this beastly torturing chest superimposed on me, and it's as if there was a demon lived there, triumphing, and extraneous to me'. Kafka was also on occasions fearful that he had been possessed and once said that, because of his illness, his body had become a bed on which 'unclean spirits' could copulate.

Lawrence had endured bad nights similar to those in Paris when he was in Port Cros. Richard Aldington remembered lying awake at night listening to his friend's 'dreadful hollow cough', and when another friend, Brigit Patmore, went to take Lawrence his breakfast, and arranged a coat round his shoulders, she noticed both how exhausted he looked and that he was bathed in perspiration. But it was bad form to suggest that anything was wrong. The person who knew most about Lawrence's bad nights was of course Frieda. She reported that his coughing was always at its worst just before dawn and how it broke her heart to hear him say, on being asked what kind of night he had passed, 'Not so bad'. On the occasion in Bandol when she responded to his request to sleep with him, she describes herself as aware all night of his 'aching inflexible chest'. There were plants in his room, a stray cat which had adopted him often slept on his bed, and the mother of the proprietor of the Beau Rivage had given him a bowl of goldfish. Never the most tactful of women, Frieda asked him why, when everything else flourished, plants and cat and goldfish, he could not do the same. 'I want to, I want to, I wish I could,' he replied. At one point in this period he told his stepdaughter how awful his nights were and confessed that 'at two in the morning, if I had a pistol I would shoot myself'.

Keats is the model in Britain of the consumptive poet. Lawrence had been an admirer of the major poems from his early youth but a book Middleton Murry published in 1925 on *Keats and Shakespeare* had, he felt, emphasized a quality in them which he called 'die away' and which he wanted to resist. Writing about the nightingales he could hear from the Villa Mirenda, he complained that their song was essentially cheerful and would never give a healthy man thoughts of what Keats in his famous ode calls 'easeful Death'. Nor would it make him dream of ceasing 'upon the midnight with no pain'. Beautiful as he felt the 'Ode to a Nightingale' was, Lawrence found something ridiculous in Keats's picture there of a world 'where men sit and hear each other groan; | Where palsy shakes a few, sad, last grey hairs'. The line which follows these, and which Lawrence does not quote, is: 'Where youth grows pale, and spectre-thin, and dies', and seems a clear reference to tuberculosis. In objecting to a certain plangent note in the ode Lawrence appears to have been fighting in himself any tendency to self-pity and defeatism; but this does not mean that he would not have shared the indignation many have felt in learning of the circumstances of Keats's death. From his medical training, and from having watched his brother die of tuberculosis, Keats would have known what was in store for him when he travelled to Rome with Joseph Severn in 1820 in order to avoid the rigours of the English winter. He had with him a bottle of laudanum and when at the beginning of 1821 his condition worsened, he asked Severn either to administer enough to terminate his sufferings or to give him the bottle. But Severn was a devout Christian and in consultation with a local English doctor, who was also fiercely opposed to suicide, removed the laudanum from the bedroom. The result was that the process of Keats's dying was far less easeful than it might have been.

Lawrence's saying that he would prefer chloroform and the long sleep to the operations Gertie Cooper chose to endure indicates that he had no ideological objections to killing himself: none of those religious scruples which in the past have led British authorities to hang failed suicides or dig up the corpses of successful ones so that they could be reburied at a crossroads with stakes driven through them. His attitude to pointless suffering is clear from his behaviour while his mother was dying from cancer. He first of all asked the doctor to hasten her end and, when this request was refused with 'you know I can't', collaborated with his sister Ada in giving Mrs Lawrence an overdose of morphine. This was a mercy-killing rather than suicide but nothing he ever wrote or said suggests that he contested the right of individuals to have mercy on themselves when their circumstances became intolerable. Maurice Magnus, a friend to whom he had been introduced by Norman Douglas, was a spendthrift who easily fell into debt. When his creditors became insistent, he fled to Malta and then poisoned himself rather than be arrested by the police. 'I like him for that,' Lawrence declared in the long biographical introduction he wrote for a memoir about his time in the French Foreign Legion which Magnus had left behind.

What circumstances are intolerable is, however, a question on which people differ a great deal and individuals who show remarkable fortitude in one context might prove surprisingly weak in another. It is nevertheless true to say that, in general, Lawrence was not someone who easily gave in. He was obviously speaking for himself as well as Gertie Cooper when he wrote to her that 'while we live we must be game. And when we come to die, we'll die game too.' The suicide of those whose circumstances seemed in no way difficult shocked him. Wealthy Americans who lived an opulent, bohemian life in Paris, Harry and Caresse Crosby were in many ways strange people for him to know. While he was staying with them in Paris, they introduced Frieda to the pleasures of the gramophone and Lawrence became so incensed with her repeated playing of Bessie Smith's *Empty Bed Blues* that he is said to have broken the record over her head. Towards the end of 1929 the Crosbys returned to America, ostensibly for the annual Harvard/Yale football game. While he was there Harry was reunited with a former mistress whom he shot before then shooting himself in what was believed to be a suicide pact. The news of this sensational event depressed Lawrence a great deal and may have occasioned the reference to a gun in his remarks to his stepdaughter about his bad nights (although the phrase is common enough). What Spenser beautifully calls 'sleep after toil, port after stormy seas' made sense for those in pain or extreme difficulty, but for a young, rich, healthy man like Crosby it seemed to Lawrence unnatural and distressing, an upsetting manifestation of what, as the 'roaring twenties' came to end, he called 'the last sort of cocktail excitement'.

It was not only pain which might have tempted Lawrence to ask for chloroform, or reach for a gun. Brigit Patmore remembered that while he was in Port Cros she had asked him why he did not write more plays. After saying that he knew he should but just did not feel very interested, he explained: 'When you think you have something in your life which makes up for everything, and then you find you haven't got it ... Two years ago I found this out.' This enigmatic remark can be interpreted as a reference to Frieda's affair with Angelo Ravagli which had begun more or less two years before. Ravagli was the husband of the woman from whom the Lawrences had rented a villa in Spotorno, a town on the Italian Riviera, soon after their final return from New Mexico in 1925. Frieda had been impressed when he made his first appearance in the full dress uniform of a lieutenant in the Italian army and their affair had begun shortly afterwards. The unhealthy closeness of Lawrence's relation with his mother had helped to give him a preternatural awareness of the feelings of others which is evident enough in his writings. It is inconceivable that he did not know about the affair and the additional meaning of Frieda's periodic visits to Germany. When he first met her, Frieda had been committed to a doctrine of free love (which he partly shared, in theory if not in practice), and since then she had not always been a model of conjugal fidelity. But one crucial difference between the early affairs and this late one was that now Lawrence was impotent and therefore in the same position with regard to Frieda as Clifford Chatterley was with regard to Connie. The way he dealt with that situation in *Lady Chatterley's Lover* suggests how difficult it would have been for him to reproach Frieda openly, but it can hardly have made him very happy.

The Magic Mountain is given philosophical weight by long disputes between Settembrini, a fervent advocate of Enlightenment values, and the Jesuit Naphta. With the arrival at the sanatorium of Peeperkorn, an elderly Dutch merchant, these two formidable debaters are thrown into the shade. Very little Peeperkorn says is coherent yet he has such a zest for life, so much animal magnetism, that he dominates and enchants Hans Castorp even though he has managed to attach to himself Frau Chauchat, the seductive Russian with whom Hans is hopelessly in love. When Peeperkorn then commits suicide it is made clear that the chief motive is sexual impotence. He is like those Turks Freud mentions at the beginning of *The Psychopathology of Everyday Life* who 'place a higher value on sexual enjoyment than on anything else, and in the event of sexual disorder . . . are plunged in a despair which contrasts strangely with their resignation towards the threat of death. One of my colleague's patients once said to him,' Freud goes on, 'Herr, you must know that if *that* comes to an end then life is of no value.' As *Lady Chatterley's Lover* makes clear, Lawrence also placed a very high value on sexual enjoyment but in Bandol he wrote 'I cannot help but be alone | for desire is dead in me, silence has grown, | and nothing now reaches out to draw | other flesh to my own.' When the painful circumstances alluded to in these lines, and the knowledge of his wife's infidelity, are added to the constant pain of his illness, it is not hard to see how there must have been a case for ending it all.

Yet suicide is hardly easy. As Dorothy Parker, who made three failed attempts, once put it, 'Razors pain you | rivers are damp | Acid stains you | and drugs cause cramp.' The degree of mental anguish has to be unimaginably great for people to ignore what the body will suffer when it is thrown out of a window or, as in the case of Virginia Woolf, voluntarily submerged under water. For those with a terminal illness who are in a position to make a calm, cost–benefit analysis of their future prospects and can therefore contemplate a relatively painless exit, there is often a banal but insoluble problem of procurement. One of the more impressive works of the French Canadian film director Denys Arcand is called *The Barbarian Invasions* and deals with a former university teacher dying of cancer. The protagonist's family and friends remove him from hospital and take him to a lakeside house in a part of the country he has always loved. They then keep him comfortable with injections of heroin until at his request they administer a fatal overdose in a moving ceremony of farewell.

The dialogue of this film is witty and the action poignant but everything is made to seem slightly unreal because the central character's son is a millionaire who can use his wealth, and entrepreneurial initiative, to solve all the practical problems of procurement which arise. Most people in his situation are not so fortunate. Despite his talk of a gun, Lawrence seems to have ruled out any similarly dramatic method for taking his own life since, with Crosby perhaps in mind, he interpolates into 'The Ship of Death' Hamlet's reference to a man making his own quietus with a 'bare bodkin' and comments:

> With daggers, bodkins, bullets, man can make
> a bruise or break an exit for his life;
> but is that a quietus, O tell me, is it quietus?

Yet had he wanted to take a less sensational route, he was in fact lucky in knowing a few people who could have given him help. His sister-in-law Else visited him in Bandol and Max Mohr, the doctor whom he had been to see in Rottach, had accompanied him there. Mohr was not only a writer who greatly admired Lawrence's work but also someone who combined extensive medical training with boldly unconventional opinions. He would have both known what Lawrence needed and been brave enough to supply it.

What suicide usually requires are not only seriously adverse circumstances but also a particular mood. From his earliest days Lawrence had been subject to periods of profound depression. In *Sons and Lovers* an exasperated Mrs Morel plumps her unaccountably tearful child down in the garden with, 'Now, cry there, Misery', and Frieda remembered this phrase when she was struggling to deal with a husband rendered almost catatonically depressed by his 'black dog'. On the whole, however, Lawrence was not a passive depressive but someone who became able to work off his black moods with outbursts of anger, often unfairly directed. He was too temperamentally active to feel defeated for long or to have agreed with the chorus in *Oepidus at Colonus* that 'not to be born is best'; and he would have appreciated the humour of the person who said that, however desirable not being born may be, very few people manage it. A wife who believed, like Ursula in *Women in Love,* that there was something not only unhealthy but immoral in being unhappy was moreover as much an influence as his mother had been on Lawrence's determination never to let depression get the better of him. Apart from which, if in his last days his sexual potency was gone, his wife was sleeping with another man, and he no longer had his health, he still had his writing.

During the war years Lawrence had said that he did not know how he could go on without his writing, and that must have been even more the case in 1929. Brigit Patmore's memory may indicate that it did not hold quite the same fascination it once did, but it still kept him absorbed. He was busy in Bandol with an attempt to interpret the symbols in *Revelation,* the last book of the Bible. In the penultimate paragraphs of this study he wrote that 'for man, as for flower and beast and bird, the supreme triumph is to be most vividly, most perfectly alive' and then: 'we ought to dance with rapture that we should be alive and in the flesh, and part of the living, incarnate cosmos.' Everyone who knew Lawrence commented on the extraordinary degree of his involvement with the natural world, how delighted and absorbed he could be by flower, beast, and bird, and all the other phenomena of the countryside. Thus in spite of the pain and discomforts of his nights, or his knowledge that Frieda was arranging another trip to Germany after Christmas (when she hoped Lawrence's sisters would be in Bandol to look after him), there was not only his writing to keep him going but also, and perhaps more importantly, the sense of still being part of the 'living, incarnate cosmos'. In his memoir *Far Away and Long Ago,* first published in 1918, W. H. Hudson wrote, 'When I hear people say that they have not found the world and life so agreeable and interesting as to be in love with it, or that they look with equanimity to its end, I am apt to think they have never been properly alive nor seen with clear vision the world they think so meanly of.' It is perhaps no accident that the man who wrote these words was a naturalist and, like Lawrence, a passionate observer of the natural world. Lawrence was not seriously prepared to kill himself because until the very last hours he never gave up hope that he would get better; he was certainly always keen not to give satisfaction to his enemies; and his writing continued to occupy and absorb him until the final week. But in addition to these reasons, there was also the fact that he never stopped loving 'life', that natural rather than social world of which he was always striving to become a more integral part.

Part II

Death

9

Andrew Morland

Although Lawrence's condition failed to improve during his second stay in Bandol, he managed to maintain a relatively active social life. In addition to Max Mohr, Frederick Carter also came to visit. He was a painter, book illustrator, and writer with a particular interest in the often baffling imagery to be found in the Book of Revelation: what *are* the seven seals, who *do* the four horsemen of the Apocalypse represent? Lawrence had been impressed by Carter's work on topics of this kind when it was first sent to him in 1923. After they had renewed contact in 1929, he invited Carter to Bandol where he stayed at the Beau Rivage during the second half of November at his host's expense. This meant that the two of them could have daily arguments about the interpretation of this or that symbol. The idea was that, by writing an introduction to a book which Carter had already completed called *The Dragon of the Alchemists*, Lawrence might help to have it published. He certainly wrote the introduction but it was because he had become increasingly dissatisfied with Carter's approach that he also, after a good deal of 'heavy' background reading, began his own short book on the Book of Revelation, and had finished it by the end of the year. The advice to people in his condition was always to rest as much as possible but however much Lawrence's illness may have restricted his physical movements, it could not stop him writing and thinking.

Another person who made an extended visit to Bandol in order to see the Lawrences was a friend from their New Mexican days, Ida Rauh. A former actress, she had been heavily involved in the socialist avant-garde to which Mabel Luhan had also been connected when both women lived in New York before and during the First World War. Ida had married the writer Max Eastman, editor at one time of the radical monthly *The Masses,* but she had left him in order to live in Taos with the painter and sculptor Andrew Dasburg, and do a little painting and sculpting herself. Lawrence had been sufficiently fond of this striking-looking woman to write a play (*David*) in which he vainly hoped she might feature. Now separated from Dasburg, Ida Rauh was travelling in Europe and must have been pleased to see people she knew well. Her presence in Bandol increased Lawrence's nostalgia for the ranch and was a constant reminder of the mostly happy days he had spent there. It was after all at the ranch that he had recovered from whatever it was that had nearly killed him in Mexico.

People such as Carter and Rauh, who paid longish visits, combined with the Brewsters to make a semi-permanent society for Lawrence; but a good number of other friends, acquaintances, or relatives passed through Bandol. He was like most people in alternating between wanting to be alone, with (although sometimes also without) Frieda; and needing to find outlets for what had certainly been in his youth a strong natural sociability. In 1926 he had written a story called 'The Man who Loved Islands' which, on a superficial level, made fun of his rich fellow writer

Compton Mackenzie for having recently acquired two of them. More fundamentally, in tracing the history of someone who moves from one sparsely populated island to another, on which there are even fewer people, and then to a third, on which there are no people at all, Lawrence was addressing himself and showing how those who try to cut themselves off completely from society (as in the past Lawrence had sometimes wanted to) must eventually go mad. But keeping up social contacts when you are gravely ill is not easy. On 23 December 1929 Lawrence was once again confined to his bed with poultices on his chest and not looking forward to the coming festivities. Why make merry when one doesn't feel merry, he said. On the following evening he nevertheless entertained a party at Beau Soleil which included the Brewsters and where he was, according to Achsah, the perfect host, serving the English Christmas specialities which his sisters had sent him and distributing inexpensive but carefully chosen presents for each guest. On New Year's Day he made what must have been the considerable and foolhardy effort to walk into the centre of Bandol in order to lunch with Ferdinando di Chiara and his American wife Anna, a couple he had first met when in Capri immediately after the war. But the wind was biting; he caught a chill; and was confined to bed once more. Tuberculosis is known as an opportunistic disease in that it tends to attack the body when it is in a weakened state; but once it is established it pays its own dues by easing the path to secondary infections. After New Year's Day, it was mostly in bed that Lawrence would have been found when he was visited in early January by Laurence Pollinger, a representative from the Curtis Brown literary agency; Edward Titus, the man responsible for publishing the cheap Paris edition of *Lady Chatterley's Lover*; and his old friend, Orioli, without whom he would hardly have been able to negotiate the first, private printing of that novel in Florence. Orioli was as usual travelling with Norman Douglas—wicked 'uncle Norman' whose fondness for adolescent boys had sent him into enforced if sybaritic exile in Italy. Douglas could never quite forgive the fact that Lawrence had twice depicted him in his writings, hinting at his sexual proclivities, and he was unfeeling in the way he made clear to others, after his visit, that of course it was obvious Lawrence was dying. Hindsight often makes poignant the way very sick people entertain hopes of recovery when in the minds of many around them they are already condemned.

In 1927 Mark Gertler had been urged by Koteliansky to write to Lawrence with advice on the best way of dealing with his illness. Although he promised that he would do so, Gertler felt it was no use unless Lawrence admitted that he had lung trouble and did not continue to pretend it was something else. He would have been confirmed in this attitude by the news of Lawrence's condition which the Huxleys had brought to London in 1929, after their failure in Paris to persuade him to have an X-ray; but that did not prevent him consulting with Koteliansky as to how best they could help. During a second brief and very recent stay at the Mundesley, which proved to be a false alarm but after which he had been forbidden to work, Gertler had met Andrew Morland, who was just beginning his time there and clearly had some interest in the arts. He and his wife Dorothy remained friendly with Gertler after he had been discharged from hospital and must have been introduced by him to Koteliansky. Because Dorothy Morland was herself suffering from tuberculosis, her husband was planning to accompany her to Menton in the South of France early in the New Year. Gertler and Koteliansky asked him whether he might not stop off to see Lawrence on the way and, after he had said that he would, wrote to Lawrence urging him to accept the visit. The fact that Lawrence agreed indicates how seriously ill he was feeling although he insisted to Gertler that it was not much use Morland coming when he was a lung doctor, and lungs were not at the root of the problem.

The Morlands arrived at the Beau Rivage on 19 January 1930 and paid a social call on the Lawrences. Frieda was out with her sister Elsa, who had recently arrived from Germany, so Lawrence entertained them on his own until she came back, impressing his visitors with how neat and quick he was in the kitchen and how rapidly tea and buns appeared. The next morning he was examined by Morland who confided to Dorothy that, although tuberculosis was certainly present, the origin of the trouble was just as much years of quasi-continuous bronchitis and that what really worried him was Lawrence's general weakness. In this period the primary resource in cases of extreme debilitation was inevitably milk. When Gertie Cooper was first preparing to go into the Mundesley Lawrence had warned her—conveying information he had gathered from Gertler—that the doctors would want to pour pint upon pint of milk down her and that she ought to say no if she found the process too sickening. According to Dorothy Morland, the difficulty in the South of France was that fresh milk was hard to come by, but she describes how she and her husband solved the problem by persuading a local farmer to tether his goat close to Lawrence's house and provide him with a regular supply. What Morland would have liked was to take Lawrence back to the Mundesley where he could himself supervise a programme of rehabilitation; but he knew from Koteliansky and Gertler how unenthusiastically such a proposal would be received and he may have thought that, in any case, the trip from Bandol to Norfolk would be too much for a man who weighed under 45 kilos. What he therefore suggested was that Lawrence should spend some time in a local sanatorium where the regime was sufficiently lax to suit his temperament and he offered to investigate what was available. Soon after leaving Bandol he wrote from Vence, the small hill town ten or so miles above Nice, and reported that he had found a sanatorium there which he thought was suitable.

Lawrence was grateful to Morland for his visit and got on particularly well with his wife, with whom he was left alone while Frieda took the doctor on sight-seeing trips. Dorothy Morland said later that he was someone who made immediate contact, cutting through the usual slow preliminaries of forming a friendship and attributed the good understanding they achieved partly to the fact that they were suffering from the same complaint, an interpretation he may well have resisted. Because her husband would not accept a fee, Lawrence promised to provide the Morlands with a signed copy of the first edition of *Lady Chatterley's Lover*. This had become an item of considerable value but it was not a present he could have given to the majority of English doctors. He liked Morland and got on well with him but that did not mean his hostility to sanatoria was still not very strong, and it is highly unlikely he would have agreed to go into one without considerable pressure from Frieda. In the past, she had always supported the decisions he had made about his own health, believing that he knew how to treat his own body better than any doctor could; but now she had a change of mind.

During Lawrence's last years, and after his death, Frieda several times described to friends, and particularly her mother, how arduous nursing him could be. It was not a role for which she was naturally well equipped. Dorothy Morland thought that her attitude was that of a large healthy woman who felt that most illnesses could be cured by a mixture of will-power, exercise, and diet, and in New Mexico Lawrence had himself once complained that she had the soul of a soldier, indelicate and robust. He said then that nobody but he could know what it was like to have her heavy German hand on him when he was sick. And yet she seems to have done her best in what were often very difficult circumstances. It may not so much have been therefore the increasing physical demands of looking after Lawrence which led her to change her mind about sanatoria, even if there might have been moments when, like the wife of Robert Louis Stevenson, she would have had to carry her husband to the toilet; but rather the increasing responsibility: a dawning sense that he might indeed finally die. This could be shared with close friends or members of her family like Else, and more especially with her daughter Barby, who had arrived in Bandol after Christmas. But Barby at this period was in a highly nervous state, having mixed in her days as an art student with friends Lawrence denounced as 'second-rate studio-arty people' and then not been able to escape what he called 'damn Bohemia', so that in the end most of the burden of care must have fallen on her mother. What may also have been relevant to Frieda's change of heart, however, is that she had planned to visit her lover Ravagli at the end of February when Lawrence's sisters were due to come to France and take over the nursing. To have her husband safely in a sanatorium by then would be even more reassuring. Yet when Frieda wrote to Ravagli to explain the situation he told her that they ought to cancel or at least postpone their arrangements because it was her duty to stay with her husband now that he was so ill. Not worrying how unfavourably this exchange might reflect on her, Frieda would later report it to others, perhaps because it endowed Ravagli with admirable, non-physical qualities which otherwise some of those others found hard to detect. Her word for the way Angelo had behaved was 'noble', which was perhaps apt, although there are signs that at this juncture Ravagli was not sure whether he wanted to continue the relationship with Frieda and that later he had to be persuaded into making it more permanent.

When Montaigne felt he was about to die, he is said to have called all his household to him and made sure that there were no wages owing to his servants and that everyone knew what legacies they could expect. Finally agreeing to go into a sanatorium was a big decision for Lawrence, and Frieda describes how he asked her to bring all his papers to his bed and grimly went through them, putting everything in order and tearing up what was no longer needed. Yet it is unlikely that this was a sign of any firm conviction that his days were numbered. Earl Brewster recorded that in all his dealings with Lawrence he never once gave the impression of doubting that he would eventually recover from his illness. Continuing to entertain hopes of recovery in January 1930 could be attributed to what Mann calls in *The Magic Mountain* 'the self-deception which marks the last stage', or to a condition which Andrew Morland was to describe in his 1932 handbook on tuberculosis: 'In advanced cases, who are near their end, the curious state known as *spes phthisica* is common: in this condition the patient tries to drive out the growing fear of death with an extreme degree of optimism.' Tolstoy has provided a dramatic account of what may be this state in his description in *Anna Karenina* of the death from tuberculosis of Levin's brother Nicholas:

> After receiving Extreme Unction the invalid suddenly felt better. He did not cough once for a whole hour, smiled, kissed Kitty's hand, thanking her with tears in his eyes, and said he felt well, had no pain, but had an appetite and felt stronger. He even sat up when they brought him some soup, and asked for a cutlet too. Hopeless as his case was, obvious as it was that he could not recover, Levin and Kitty were for that hour both in the same state of excitement, happy yet timid and fearful of being mistaken.

Lawrence may have been unreasonably optimistic about his future prospects but the optimism he displayed was guarded and unlike Nicholas (whose case may be complicated by extreme unction) he was not yet quite on his deathbed. A more likely explanation of his refusal to accept he was dying than *spes phthisica*, therefore, is that he had managed narrowly to escape death so many times before. His experience as an adolescent and as a young schoolteacher, together with his many narrow escapes subsequently (including the one from the deadly influenza of 1919 which had seen off so many millions of his contemporaries), would have made him a firm believer in that defiant protest of folk wisdom against the cold-blooded actuaries: 'The creaking door hangs longest.' It was after settling his affairs in Bandol that he sent Barby to Toulon in order to make enquiries about visas so that they could all three of them (Frieda, Barby, and himself) go back to New Mexico. The Americans would not have given him a visa without a medical inspection and the likelihood of his again being able to talk himself past a doctor, as he had in El Paso, was nil; but with Ida Rauh in the vicinity he dreamt of New Mexico nonetheless. Wanting to go there was unlikely to have been *spes phthisica* but rather the urge he had always had, when things were not going well in one place, to move rapidly on to another. During the war years when the British authorities refused to grant him a passport which would allow him to emigrate to the United States and when his known opposition to the war, and German wife, then led them to insist that he should move inland, out of the Cornish cottage he was renting and away from the sea, he had felt horribly trapped and hemmed in. Once hostilities had ceased and it became possible to leave Britain, he became a great traveller and someone who always felt, or at least hoped, that there was a happier and healthier life elsewhere. This was certainly one Lawrence but there was also another who could write in a review published in 1927: 'We travel, perhaps, with a secret and absurd hope of setting foot on the Hesperides, or running our boat up a little creek and landing in the Garden of Eden. The hope is always defeated. There is no Garden of Eden, and the Hesperides never were.'

10

Ad Astra

Being such a great traveller meant that Lawrence had covered during his lifetime vast distances in Australia, the United States, and Mexico. Quite often the means of transport at his disposal were primitive and on occasions his routes were also dangerous. Because he was so ill, his worst journey had perhaps been the long way back from Oaxaca to Mexico City on a railway line which had frequently been cut during the recent civil war and past stations pock-marked with bullets. But now, on 5 February 1930, the short and peaceful trip between Bandol and Nice, not much more that a hundred miles long, proved almost as bad. The main trouble was that, after being driven to Toulon station, he needed all the help Frieda and Earl Brewster could give him to negotiate the flights of steps between the platforms. Barby had arranged that a friend of hers from art school, Blair Hughes-Stanton, should meet them at Nice with his car. This made the final leg of the journey up the narrow winding roads to Vence more comfortable but it still meant that, when they arrived at the Ad Astra sanatorium, Hughes-Stanton had to carry an exhausted Lawrence into the building.

Ad Astra was not the most encouraging name for a sanatorium, all of whose occupants would be anxious about their next port of call. It derived from images of the sun, moon, and stars which decorated the building's outside walls. These were rumoured to be the result of it having once been owned or rented by Camille Flammarion, a leading French astronomer and the author of an immensely popular work of science fiction, *The End of the World* (1893), which pre-dates H. G. Wells's *War of the Worlds* by five years. The heavenly bodies on its exterior were the most flamboyant features of the Ad Astra which otherwise operated like a hotel with discreet medical supervision. There may have been reasons for this in the attitude of the local authorities. In an official guide available throughout the 1930s the visitor is warned that the Vence climate is totally unsuitable for those with tuberculosis and that they will always find their condition worsened by 'a stay in our town'. In case this message was not clear enough, the authors of the guide (issued by the *Syndicat d'Initiative*) go on later to combat the rumour that Vence was full of sick people and to suggest that it was being spread by malicious and envious competitors. They pointed out that there were only two sanatoria in the town, both a long way from the main square and there was therefore much less chance of catching tuberculosis in Vence than there would be in Paris where one of the main hospitals for the disease was only separated from the general public by the width of a road. Like the man Freud describes who indignantly denied that he had taken someone's kettle but added that in any case it had a hole in it, they then said that, in their view, tuberculosis was not really catchable but rather 'a family disease, only contagious through immediate and prolonged contact in childhood'. There were fortunes to be made in looking after sufferers from tuberculosis and many of the Alpine resorts seemed to have been able to cater for both those who were sick and healthy skiers on holiday. But it is clear from the guide book that the Vence authorities were attempting to attract to their town retired French 'colonials'—people who had spent their working lives in hot countries—and they appeared to have felt that this aim was not consistent with catering for consumptives.

Had Lawrence been able to read the guide book he might have been reminded of an unpleasant incident in June 1928 when he and Frieda were travelling in France with the Brewsters and found a hotel at St Nizier, not far from Grenoble, which all agreed was perfect. But the next morning the proprietor came to the Brewsters and told them that Lawrence would have to leave because he had coughed so much during the night. Everyone pretended that they had changed their minds about the hotel which was not, they now decided, as ideal as they had first thought. Although Lawrence said nothing at the time, he was fully aware of what had happened. He may in company have done all he could to minimize the importance of his frequent coughing and spitting but he understood their effect on others, once complaining that he coughed 'to the general annoyance and cold commiseration of a nervous universe'. When Chekhov arrived in the German spa where he was soon to die, he was asked to leave the first hotel he found there after only two days because his coughing during the night disturbed the other guests. In his case, as in Lawrence's, the objection may have been a straightforwardly commercial one; but it may also have been mixed with the prejudice, ignorance, and fear that often conditioned the general attitude to tuberculosis at this time. It is hard to tell whether the authorities in Vence were affected by this prejudice and fear (ignorant of tuberculosis they clearly show they were), or whether they were simply trying to make hard-headed decisions about the kind of tourist resort, or retirement centre, they wanted to develop.

A small walled town on a hill, with some buildings which date back to the middle ages, Vence is delightfully picturesque and must have been particularly so in 1930 when the surrounding countryside was not yet littered with villas, hotels, and apartment blocks. But its many attractions were ones Lawrence never had the opportunity to explore, or even see. The Ad Astra is now no more but it then stood some three or four hundred yards outside the town wall on the road south to St Paul. He was given a room on the top, fourth floor with a balcony and a sight of the sea at Cagnes-sur-mer which was where, after more than a week in a Vence hotel, Frieda went with Barby to stay in a villa the di Chiaras had just vacated. Having a view of the sea pleased Lawrence, as did the mimosa which was everywhere in bloom and reminded him of his days in Australia. When he first arrived he praised the quality of the air and felt it did him good. Although the importance of air quality in the treatment of tuberculosis was largely mythical, one of the reasons the Vence authorities might have been fearful of their town becoming a haven for consumptives was that it stands 325 metres above sea level and might therefore have been thought to combine the benefits of a Mediterranean climate with just a few of those to be found in the Alpine resorts.

As much as he liked the view which his balcony offered, and appreciated the air which he could breathe in from it, a major drawback of the Ad Astra for Lawrence was that it had no lift. To eat with the other patients he had to go down (and then back up again) two flights of steep stairs and perhaps as a result he increasingly had meals brought to his room. Given how little he was able to eat, this may not have seemed very important but it meant that he was more alone than he might have been and never got to know any of his fellow sufferers. When he had moved from a chalet in the mountains near Gsteig to the building Aldington had borrowed at the summit of a steep hill on the island of Port Cros, he had complained that he was always being 'perched'. Now he felt perched once again, and isolated. In their vivid, detailed accounts of sanatorium life, both Thomas Mann and Derek Lindsay emphasize how quickly those suffering from tuberculosis were able to bond together and form their own special world with its own rules and values. Mann in particular had reservations about this phenomenon but it clearly brought relief and satisfaction to its participants cut off and in a sense rejected as they were by what is known as the real world. Lawrence was perhaps too ill to join whatever society of this kind had formed in the Ad Astra but there was in any case an entry fee he might have felt either reluctant or not in a position to pay. Mann and Lindsay's characters bond together so easily because they freely acknowledge that the TB bacillus is threatening or ruining their lives, just as it had threatened or ruined the lives of hundreds of thousands of others elsewhere. They accept that they are consumptive and draw strength from the company of those who have also accepted that they belong to the same, often vilified group.

The Ad Astra was run by two doctors called Pouymayou and Madinier. It was Madinier who took charge of Lawrence, examining and having him X-rayed shortly after he arrived. The results were reported to Morland in a letter from Madinier which included a sketch of Lawrence's lungs. This showed that there were lesions or cavities at the apex of both. The only hope, Morland's French colleague wrote, was that these lesions were not recent, something which could not be determined from an X-ray. What particularly worried him, however, apart from the frequent coughing and expectoration, was his patient's general run-down condition (his 'état de profonde déchéance organique'). It was presumably by Madinier that Barby was told that tuberculosis had reached Lawrence's intestines, as it did Chekhov's. Palliative care seemed the only option and hence the same camphor oil injections Chekhov had received in his final days. What is interesting about these in Lawrence's case is that they went directly into the legs ('I want my legs back again', he had written to Emily's daughter Margaret on 2 February, just before going to Vence). He himself did not know or believe that Madinier regarded his condition as critical and though, in his first extant use of the word in relation to himself, he talked of some 'slight tubercular trouble', he gave no sign of believing that this mattered much. 'But the broncs are awful', he wrote to Maria Huxley, 'and they have inflamed my lower man, the *ventre* and the liver.'

Andrew Morland had told Lawrence that if he wanted to get better he had to do absolutely nothing, make no attempts at exercise and that he should 'do *no* work, see *no* people, and not even think'. This was the standard first move in all sanatorium treatment and it could last a long time: when Morland was wondering whether it might after all be possible to get Lawrence to the Mundesley, and realized that he himself was shortly going to have to be away from the sanatorium for a considerable period, he told Gertler that it would not much matter because there was little likelihood of Lawrence being able to leave his room 'for several months'. One point of confining him to his room would have been to free him from all the supposed stresses and excitements of his profession as a writer. The attitude of those in charge at the Ad Astra was less draconian so that, while Lawrence was there, he not only read a good deal but began a review of a book of essays on art and religion by the English printmaker and sculptor Eric Gill. Lawrence was an excellent reviewer who provided his readers with clear, conscientious descriptions of the books under consideration while at the same time conveying his own opinion of them in what were always forcible and sometimes witty terms. His views on Gill are the last words he wrote for the general public but it is impossible to detect in them any sign of decreasing intellectual energy. There is perhaps, on the contrary, rather too much energy as, in the first part of the review ('Let us say all the bad things first'), he pitches into Gill for his lack of skill as a writer and his inadequate ratiocinative powers. 'A crude and crass amateur' is what Lawrence feels he is in these two departments and he justifies the unkindness of the second adjective by complaining that the manner in which Gill writes is 'maddening, like a tiresome uneducated workman arguing in a pub—*argefying* would be a better word—and banging his fists'. He himself was very far from being uneducated but since his own polemical manner usually consists of stating a position and then stating it again and again, with numerous qualifications and stylistic variations, he can sometimes make his readers feel that they are on the losing end of a pub argument with no time to draw breath before the fist comes thumping down on the bar once again. He is, however, nearly always precise and concrete whereas he is able to quote short passages from Gill's book which illustrate the kind of fondness for abstract terms that makes it hard to work out what someone wants to say.

When Lawrence comes to discuss 'the good side' of Gill's book, he focuses on an essay entitled 'Slavery and Freedom' and what he calls the great and invaluable truth of the claim he finds in it. This is that slavery consists in a man doing what he likes in his spare time while doing what is required of him during his working hours whereas, in a state of freedom, the reverse is true. The state of slavery can only exist, according to Gill, when what men like to do is please themselves whereas freedom depends on men wanting to please God. Lawrence spends the rest of his review trying to tease out what 'pleasing God' might mean and in the process arrives at a definition of the second term which he assumes Gill would share. This is despite his having asked why people keep on trying to define words 'like Art, Beauty and God, words which represent deep emotional states in us, and are therefore incapable of definition'. The same contradiction occurs in his last poems, in one of which ('Tabernacle') he says that anyone trying to ascribe attributes to God, or to oblivion, ought to be cast out because 'God is a deeper forgetting far than sleep | and all description is a blasphemy'. Yet another poem is called 'The Body of God' and includes the beautiful and characteristic 'There is no god | apart from poppies and the flying fish | men singing songs, and women brushing their hair in the sun'.

What is implied by Gill's phrase 'Pleasing God', Lawrence writes, is only 'happily doing one's best at the job in hand, and being livingly absorbed in an activity which makes one in touch with the heart of all things—call it God. It is a state of absorption into the creative spirit, which is God.' What he feels certain of is that God is not the moralistic, judging figure of orthodox religion but rather the power which 'enters us and imbues us with his strength and glory and might and honour and beauty and wisdom'. He goes on:

> The workman making a pair of shoes with happy absorption in skill is imbued with the god of strength and honour and beauty, undeniable. Happy, intense absorption in any work, which is to be brought as near to perfection as possible, this is a state of being with God, and the men who have not known it have missed life itself.

All those who knew Lawrence commented on his remarkable ability to become completely absorbed not only in his writing, which he could carry on in a room where people around him were talking, or in his painting, but also in the most menial of household tasks. Although therefore he was still only 44 and about to die, there was no sense in which, by these criteria, he could be said to have missed out on life.

Lawrence wrote over two thousand words of the Gill review but, after a couple of weeks of sanatorium life, he had become so sick and was in such frequent, acute pain that Frieda dissuaded him from finishing it. For the whole of his time at the Ad Astra a temperature chart survives, conscientiously filled in and signed by the same nurse. It shows that for the first two weeks he usually had a morning temperature of 36.5 which went up to 37.5 in the evening but that from 20 February onwards it tended to stay at or below 37 except for a sudden surge towards 38 on the day before he was preparing to leave. This is surprising in that it was from about the 20th that his condition worsened dramatically in what may or may not have been a natural development of his disease. It was Morland who later said that Lawrence developed pleurisy while at the Ad Astra, and certainly pleurisy is notorious for causing acute pain with each breath. But quite why his pleura had become inflamed is now impossible to say. It may be that the prejudice of his working-class background was confirmed and he had picked up an infection which was lurking in the sanatorium itself; but if this was the case, it is perhaps strange to find no obvious sign of it in his temperature chart.

In addition to the camphor oil injections, Lawrence was given one tablet at six in the evening, and another at midnight, of a preparation which contained codeine. This was the weakest of the three opium-derived drugs administered to those in Lawrence's condition. Next in strength was morphine, which he seems to have refused until the last day of his life, and then heroin (in his 1932 handbook Andrew Morland insisted that, in the final stages of tuberculosis, there was 'no drug to equal heroin'). The codeine does not seem to have done much good. One evening when Frieda was about to leave him and return to Cagnes, Lawrence told her that he would have to fight several battles of Waterloo before the following morning. A day or so later he asked her to spend the night in his room and she therefore passed twelve uncomfortable hours on a cane chair, listening to her husband's sufferings but unable to do anything about them. It depressed her that there were no stars in the sky to distract her from the sound which came from young and old coughing in so many different rooms. The only satisfaction the coughers could have had was that this was a hotel no one would ask them to leave. Although he was never keen to advertise the fact, Lawrence wore glasses to read and he was also a little deaf. Frieda was relieved that this second minor infirmity meant that he did not seem to hear the young girl from the next room who cried out in her despair, 'Mama, mama, je souffre tant'. It must have been after this experience that Frieda decided to take a room in the Ad Astra itself. She was there from the 22nd and ended up with a bill for just over 1,000 francs or around 10 pounds.

Lawrence's strong tendency to blame his own sufferings on their context now made itself felt so that, after initially quite liking the Ad Astra, it became a 'beastly place' and he urged Frieda to move him elsewhere. When he first arrived he had appreciated the fact that the only sign of the Ad Astra being a sanatorium was that a nurse recorded his temperature every morning and evening, and that he was examined by the doctors once a week. Now that he was so ill he failed to see the point of being there when those in charge had no solutions to offer apart from camphor oil, codeine, and the small amount of digitalis he seems to have been given in his last week. Finding somewhere to go which was nearby was, however, a difficult task for Frieda to perform at short notice especially as, according to Barby, the residents of Vence—who may have read their own town guide—seemed terrified of renting their houses to someone with Lawrence's complaint and in his condition. But eventually Frieda found a villa which was outside the walls and on the opposite side of the town. An indication that she felt Lawrence was now even sicker than he had been after his major haemorrhage in the Villa Mirenda is that she hired a nurse in Nice (probably from an agency Morland had suggested), as well as arranging that a local Corsican doctor, Dr Maestracci, should be on hand after she had brought Lawrence 'home'. Through no particular fault of its own, the Ad Astra had fulfilled the worst fears of a man always hostile to sanatoria. 'This place no good' he was to write to both Dorothy Morland and Maria Huxley just before he left.

11

Visitors

Western society imposes numerous obligations on the very sick or dying, one of which is the willingness to receive visitors: if Katherine Mansfield had really refused to see Middleton Murry, her 'Keep that bugger away from me' would have required considerable psychological as well as physical effort. The obligation to receive final visits is of course much less strong now than it was in previous centuries when the long stream through the bedroom of those determined to say their last farewell was an accepted feature of social life. Death was a drama in which the dying were expected to play their proper part. One of the best implicit judgements on the role played by visitors is said to have been made by the dying Disraeli who asked his intimates to try and keep Queen Victoria away. This was because, he claimed, all she would want him to do was carry a message to her dear departed Albert.

How many visitors appeared depended on who you were but also on whether or not people died at home, surrounded by all their friends and relatives in the days when spending all one's life in the same place was the rule rather than the exception. Lawrence was far in Vence from anything which could be described as his own home yet, before she took a room at the Ad Astra, Frieda tried to suggest that nothing much had changed since Bandol by visiting him every day, usually in the company of his stepdaughter. The same impression was also fostered by occasional visits from Ida Rauh, who had preceded the Lawrences to the Vence area in order perhaps to link up with Emma Goldman, an old friend from her New York days who had been deported from the United States for her anarchist activities and was at that time living in or near Nice. Towards the end of Lawrence's stay in the sanatorium, Aldous and Maria Huxley appeared. Having been in London for the short run of a play entitled *This Way to Paradise*, they were looking for a house to rent in the South of France but had returned to Vence principally because they were anxious about Lawrence's state. The play was a stage adaptation by a now forgotten writer called Campbell Dixon of Aldous's recent *Point Counter Point* (1928), a novel which had upset Lawrence because it contained a very obvious portrait of himself. He appeared under the name of Mark Rampion, a writer and painter of working-class origins with a well-born wife. It may have galled Lawrence as he lay in the Ad Astra to realize that now Rampion could not only be read about between the covers of Huxley's book but was treading the boards in London and widely regarded as the most successful element in an otherwise coolly received production. Am I really such a gas-bag and such a bore, he had complained when he first read the novel, and he said then that the portrait made him feel like a badger with a hole on Wimbledon Common, trying not to be caught. To one of the short poems he called 'Pansies', chiefly because of the derivation of that English word from *pensées*, he gave the title 'I am in a novel', and he commented that 'If this is what Archibald thinks of me | he sure thinks a lot of lies'. There are many ways in which Rampion does give a superficial and inaccurate impression of what Lawrence was like, but the character is nevertheless treated warmly. He is a far more sympathetic figure than, for example, Lawrence's roughly contemporary depiction of Huxley in *Lady Chatterley's Lover* as Hammond, one of the group of intellectuals who indulge in cynical and disillusioned discussions of sex at Wragby Hall and a man who is described at one point as 'more closely connected with his typewriter' than his wife. Whether or not he recognized this difference, Lawrence's anger died down after a while as he reminded himself that, whatever Aldous wrote, he was always good company and a loyal friend ('*Poor* old Aldous, *poor* old Aldous', he was once heard to mutter as he pondered Huxley's intensely cerebral nature). He would have been glad to see him again and especially glad to see Maria. She had formerly been Maria Nys, the daughter of a Belgian industrialist who had sent her to England during the war into the safe-keeping of Lady Ottoline Morrell and Lawrence had probably known her longer than he had known her husband.

These visitors were not of the kind which required any great social effort from a Lawrence whom Huxley described as now 'such a miserable wreck of himself and suffering so much pain'. He was largely protected from the other kind by his location although in 1930 the Côte d'Azur was as full of English residents as the Dordogne is now, and many of them were painters or writers. On the coast within easy visiting distance, for instance, was Cap Ferrat where Somerset Maugham had recently bought a villa and where he lavishly entertained other artists as well as rich aristocrats and celebrities from the worlds of finance and politics. His own history of tuberculosis might have made him a likely visitor but he and Lawrence had already met in Mexico in 1924 and not hit it off.

Their contacts had failed to dispel Lawrence's prejudice that Maugham was a 'narrow-gutted "artist" with a stutter', and nor did they prevent Maugham from later describing Lawrence as 'a sick man of abnormal irritability, whose nature was warped by poverty and cankered with a rankling envy'. A visit to Vence would have been an act of hypocrisy for one party and a trial for the other.

A member of the group with which Maugham liked to mingle—those who comprised what would now be called the Côte d'Azur's jet set—was the Aga Khan. He had met Frieda in London in the summer of 1929 at the time of the exhibition of Lawrence's paintings. Arriving to view them just after the police had closed the exhibition down and turned thirteen paintings to the wall, he was able to use his prestige to have them all turned round again for his benefit and that of an anonymous visitor from Nottingham who happened also to be in the room. Later he dined with Frieda and must have expressed his admiration for what he had seen. His visit to Vence was as much a question of business as sympathy since he had a plan for showing the pictures in a private gallery in Paris; but Lawrence was cheered by it and thought the Aga Khan and his wife 'very nice'. Whatever 'rankling envy' Lawrence may have suffered from (and there is certainly very little sign of any), it did not extend to all aristocrats or all members of England's upper crust. He had been very friendly with Lady Ottoline Morrell and perhaps even more so with Cynthia Asquith who was the daughter of a lord and, when he first met her, the daughter-in-law of the prime minister. Being a miner's son with an ineradicable Midlands' accent did not prevent him quickly overcoming any initial unease which contact with the well born might have brought, and being able to establish warm and easy relations with those among them whom he found sympathetic and intelligent. It helped that the well born in question were usually in awe of his talents, but it may also have helped his sense of his own relation to them that he himself was married to an aristocrat, even if a very minor one; and even also if Frieda's family name of von Richthofen had become well known only because of the exploits during the war of her distant cousin Manfred, the daring fighter pilot known throughout Europe as 'the red baron'.

The Aga Khan and his wife came to Vence on 27 February, four days after a visit from H. G. Wells, who was then living in the nearby town of Grasse with Odette Keun, the latest in a long line of mistresses. Lawrence had first been introduced to Wells in November 1909 and must then have been excited to meet a man he admired so much, not for his science fiction but for novels of 'ordinary' life such as *Love and Mr Lewisham*, *Kipps*, and above all *Tono-Bungay*, which had just been serialized in the recently launched *English Review*, edited by Ford Madox Ford (or Ford Madox Hueffer as he was at that time called). It was about the period of this meeting that he confidently told Jessie Chambers that he expected eventually to earn the massive sum of £2,000 a year through his writing. The older man was certainly someone to be admired because of the books he had written but he was also a role model for Lawrence in that he had demonstrated how spectacularly someone from a modest background could—in the phrase Mrs Lawrence was fond of using—'get on'. When he died in 1946 Wells left £60,000, having previously lived (according to Rebecca West) like minor royalty.

Partly because Wells was almost twenty years older than Lawrence, there were crucial differences as well as strong similarities between them. Both their backgrounds could fairly be described as 'working class' but whereas, as a miner, Arthur Lawrence was a fully paid-up member of the industrial proletariat, the father of Wells began his working life as a gardener on a large country estate. He then became a very unsuccessful shopkeeper in Bromley, augmenting his meagre income by playing cricket for Kent (Lawrence must have remembered this unusual detail when, in the second version of *Lady Chatterley's Lover,* he made the figure we now know as Mellors the son of a professional cricketer). The mothers of both men were women with social aspirations, dissatisfied with their husbands. Mrs Wells had been a housekeeper on a reasonably grand scale and derived her own view of how life should be lived from the people she served. She scraped together enough money to send her gifted son to an inadequate but nonetheless private elementary school. Like Lawrence, Wells was somewhat weedy as a child and in adolescence and young manhood he had several haemorrhages which suggested tuberculosis. It was after one of these that, again like Lawrence, he gave up teaching and decided he would try to earn his living through writing. The first (and best) novels he then wrote were strongly autobiographical and he preceded Lawrence in handling topics which in his time were regarded as shocking. Published in the same year as *Tono-Bungay,* for example, was *Ann Veronica,* a novel partly based on Wells's experience of leaving his wife in order to 'live in sin' with another woman. This was rejected by Macmillan, his usual publisher, on the grounds that it would cause a scandal. Given difficulties of a similar nature which Lawrence was later to experience, there is some irony in his having asked Edward Garnett whether his own second novel

(*The Trespasser*) was really erotic, as Ford Madox Ford had suggested, and his then having added that he would not like to be talked about 'in an *Ann Veronica* fashion'.

Lawrence lost touch with Wells during the war and for a long time afterwards, although he would have heard of him from his friend Rebecca West, who was for several years one of Odette Keun's predecessors. Both authors wrote fictions in the 1920s which were simultaneously tracts for good, non-democratic government; and they would have agreed that the world needed to be run by a small body of competent people, an oligarchy of those of intellectual and moral distinction (with in Lawrence's case an emphasis on 'moral' which quickly shades off into the spiritual). But a good deal of Wells's time was also spent on a massive *Outline of History* (abbreviated a little later into *A Short History of the World)*, and its successor *The Science of Life*, for which he had recruited Julian Huxley. These were works of what the French call *haute vulgarisation* and they made him a lot of money. The first, apparently fictional consequence of his move to Grasse with Odette Keun was the appearance in 1926 of volume one of *The World of William Clissold*, which Lawrence reviewed and which he found very disappointing. 'A sexagenarian bore' is how he describes its narrator Clissold, complaining that the supposed novel in which he appeared was just an excuse for Wells to unload his by now familiar ideas on religion, science, and politics. The scene was set in a villa in a southern French town which is obviously Grasse where Clissold is living with a woman much younger than himself who admires him above all for his mind, and it is the celebration of that attribute in the book which brings out a fundamental difference between Wells and his reviewer. Clissold explains that his mental activities have always been more important to him than any others but, Lawrence asked, since even he admits that thoughts must always be preceded by 'by some obscure physical happenings', why cannot he see that the mind itself is dependent on a 'full and subtle emotional life'?

At the end of his review, Lawrence said that he hoped for better things from volumes two and three of *The World of William Clissold* given that in the past the man who was promising to produce them had written 'such brilliant and such very genuine novels'. If this was meant to mollify, it would have cut no ice with Wells but then neither would he have been much disturbed by sharp criticism from a man like Lawrence. He was used to hostile remarks (his close friend Shaw told him that in *Clissold* he had forgotten he was a novelist), and he rarely allowed them to affect his social relations with other writers. When Julian Huxley and his wife came to stay with him at Grasse in 1928, they would have given him news of the Lawrences because they had stopped off to see them in Bandol on the way. Wells had loyally put his name down for a copy of *Lady Chatterley's Lover* and wrote to Lawrence when some hitch prevented it from arriving. It is likely to have been to this letter that Frieda was responding when she wrote from the Ad Astra in February 1930 and said that it had pleased her husband to have heard from Wells. It was she who suggested he should visit Lawrence ('if he hasn't had a bad day!'), and she then added: 'I am worried about Lorenzo & the only thing I can think of for him is a journey on a big yacht.' This was almost certainly a hint to a person Frieda must have felt was rich enough to take it up, but although Wells ignored the reference to the yacht he did take the short drive over to Vence. 'A common temporary soul' was

Lawrence's judgement on a man who, when he had first met him, was healthy and prosperous and who now, at 63, must have seemed equally healthy to his desperately sick observer, and who was certainly richer. Wells's judgement on Lawrence was much more surprising. Everyone else who saw him was immediately alarmed by his emaciated state but Wells took the view that Lawrence was nowhere near as ill as he and others thought, and that the problem was chiefly a question of hysteria.

This diagnosis was recorded by Barby but there is confirmation for it in the memories of an American sculptor called Jo Davidson who was visiting Grasse at the time. He specialized in busts of famous people and Wells had very recently been one of his subjects. Sitting for Davidson had been something Wells enjoyed so he urged him to go and see Lawrence on the grounds that the latter's troubles were largely mental and having a sculpture made of him might lift his spirits. Davidson and his wife arrived at the Ad Astra on 26 February and found Lawrence having lunch on his balcony. There was talk of mutual friends (Davidson and Ida Rauh were distantly related through marriage), and he invited Lawrence, who had expressed a distaste for plasticine, to feel the cool clean clay he was using. After an hour Lawrence sent him down the steep stairs to find something to eat and, when he came back, his subject was in bed. He requested to stay there for the rest of the session which, he later complained, tired him out a great deal. Davidson was so far from sharing Wells's view of Lawrence's condition that, when he returned to Paris, he told his compatriot Mrs Harry Payne Whitney (a Vanderbilt before her marriage) how desperately ill he was. In the great tradition of American philanthropy, she asked him to phone Frieda with an offer to cover any medical expenses which might be required but by then it was too late.

Davidson's visit to Lawrence was criticized later when there was wholly inaccurate talk of his having 'burst into the sickroom'. It seemed wrong to some that he should have been modelling a bust only four days before the death of its subject. These complaints are at variance with what had been, until at least the end of the nineteenth century, a strong morbid curiosity as to how people looked at the time of their death. This expressed itself most obviously in the fashion for the death mask. William James is said to have derived comfort from contemplating the death mask of Pascal and in the nineteenth century it was fashionable to buy a copy of the death mask of Keats, which you could hang up by a nail on the wall. The moulds for these masks were of course taken after the subjects were dead but the process could be intrusive, and almost as shocking therefore as Davidson's visit was considered by some to be. This was because the taking of the mould often needed to be done very quickly after death in order to avoid the risks of decomposition. It is now well known, for example, that the death mask of Balzac available in the nineteenth century is a fake because, by the time the workmen arrived with their plaster, decomposition had set in and his nose had (in the words of one commentator) run into the sheets. Maupassant records how startled he was when he was presented with a plaster cast of Flaubert and saw that it came with real eyebrows, uprooted as the plaster came off the face. Accidents like this were avoided once the making of death masks began to be replaced by the fashion for taking photographs of corpses as they lay on their deathbeds. Both practices now seem macabre and Davidson may have felt later that there was something macabre in his visit to Lawrence although the main charge against him was presumably that he had taken the likeness of a dying not a dead subject, and that (as it were) he could not be bothered to wait. Yet if there was any blame in the matter it belonged to Wells rather than to him. Lawrence judged the clay model which Davidson made mediocre and, cast in bronze, it certainly looks mediocre now, and much less striking than several photographs of him in his last years, which reveal how painfully thin and gaunt he had become (a comparison which is perhaps also macabre). After Lawrence had died, Frieda was either old-fashioned or unsentimental enough to regret that there had been neither the time nor the facilities to have a death mask made.

12

The Hour of Our Death

'Sudden death, the only thing to fear' is one of Pascal's better-known *pensées*. Nowadays our attitude is likely to be different. Most of us would declare a preference for dropping dead in the street rather than dying from a long and painful illness. Christians in the past feared sudden death because it left them no time to confess their sins and settle their spiritual as well as material affairs. This was why in the nineteenth century tuberculosis was sometime regarded as a good disease to have, and why it was so often associated with the 'good' or exemplary deaths recorded in the religious journals. There was little chance of it creeping up unawares and there were usually plenty of warning signs before it became life-threatening. It was a disease which gave its victims time to prepare for death and become reconciled to it. Yet when on 1 March 1930 Lawrence angrily discharged himself from the Ad Astra, he was probably not at all reconciled to dying but rather expecting that he was in for one of those hard battles from which he had emerged victorious so many times before. 'I can't die,' Frieda had remembered him saying, 'I can't die, I hate them too much! I have given too much and what did I get in return?'

The house which Frieda had rented was known as the Villa Robermond, presumably after its owners (past or present), and not at all equipped for nursing the dying. While he was still in the Ad Astra, Lawrence allowed his wife to put on his shoes for him for the first time in their life together, and she had a memory of an uncomfortable journey in a 'shaking' taxi from the sanatorium to the other side of town. Barby recalled seeing her mother and stepfather arriving at the rented villa and Lawrence staggering up the few steps of the veranda with the help of the chauffeur, declaring that he was very ill. He went to bed immediately and Frieda then called the Corsican doctor to examine him. When he emerged from the bedroom, Dr Maestracci declared there was little hope but urged the others not to communicate this impression to Lawrence.

The bed to which Lawrence immediately retired, Frieda made a point of remarking, was shortly to be his deathbed. There is a memorable deathbed scene at the beginning of John Donne's great poem, 'A Valediction: Forbidding Mourning':

> As virtuous men pass mildly away,
> And whisper to their souls, to go,
> While some of their sad friends do say,
> The breath goes now, and some say, no:

Donne's purpose in evoking this definitive parting is to compare it with a temporary one forced on a loving husband and wife by circumstances and his idealization of death therefore occurs in a context which is gently ironic. It would be comforting but unreasonable to assume that the virtue of a man ensures that he can pass away mildly and only has to whisper instructions to his soul to leave the body: that there is no discomfort involved in giving up the ghost. Implicit in the reference to the friends who surround the dying is the assumption that death is a public event and this is largely what it remained from Donne's time until the twentieth century. Although it did not occur in a hospital, the death of Lawrence was on the other hand a more recognizably modern, private death with a limited number of onlookers. With nothing much else to do, Barby had stayed on in Bandol to help Frieda. The youngest of Frieda's three children by Ernest Weekley, she had been the first to rebel against the hostile view of her mother with which she had been indoctrinated. When Frieda decided to leave home in order to live with Lawrence it must have been a great shock to Barby and her two siblings, as it certainly was to Weekley himself who later complained that the public shame of the ensuing divorce ruined any chance he might have had of finding a post in Oxbridge. He was able to impose a legal ban on Frieda ever seeing her children again without his permission, while they remained minors (half-yearly visits were what he eventually allowed). All three later re-established good relations with their mother but it was Barby, the most artistic as well as the most unsettled, who defied most obviously her Weekley background and developed a strong bond with her stepfather. Affection for Lawrence as well as the desire to support her mother was therefore what had kept her in Bandol and brought her to Vence. After his death, when her mental state deteriorated rapidly, she would lie outside what had been his bedroom, banging her head against the door and crying out like King Lear 'Nothing, nothing, nothing'.

Earl Brewster had accompanied Lawrence to Vence but had then taken an opportunity which had arisen for him to go back to India for a short while because he did not suspect that his friend's death was imminent. Had they known the situation was so serious, one or other of Lawrence's two sisters would certainly have rushed out to see him but a fortnight previously he had written to the elder, Emily, in order to prevent that happening. He had described himself then as in slow but not sudden danger and said that, although he would have to take care, there was no need for either her or Ada to worry. On 1 March, therefore, Frieda and Barby were probably alone in the Villa Robermond except that there was now professional help on hand in the form of the hired nurse. Who she was is difficult to say. She may have been called Evelyn Thorogood since in October 1937 someone calling herself by that name sent to the *Evening Standard* a page of doodles which she claimed to have found 'one morning on [Lawrence's] breakfast tray', but which are demonstrably not his. The newspaper was at that time running a series on doodles—those attributed to Lawrence shared a page with six other sets—and paid half a guinea to any person who sent in a set which was deemed publishable. For the most interesting doodles of the week, there was also a prize of 10 guineas, which Evelyn Thorogood did not win. She may nevertheless have been Lawrence's nurse and confused the drawings with those made by another patient in the South of France whom she had been hired to attend. Whether or not she was is of only minor importance because Lawrence took an immediate dislike to her and refused to notice her presence, with the result that she counts little in the story of his final hours. Since Barby describes the nurse as inoffensive and unobtrusive, it may be that what he was really refusing was any acknowledgement of what her presence signified. Hiring a nurse was a much more common practice then than it is now but this was because so many more people died at home and professional help was often considered appropriate and necessary for the final stages. Except in wealthy households, seeing a hired nurse come into your bedroom would not have been a good omen.

By claiming in the note she sent to the *Evening Standard* that she had found the doodles on Lawrence's breakfast tray 'one morning', Evelyn Thorogood implies that there were many more; but in fact one morning in the Villa Robermond was all he had. On the evening of 1 March Frieda went to sleep on a couch in Lawrence's bedroom where he could see her and on the 2nd he was sufficiently well to get up long enough to brush his teeth. Barby cooked his lunch and when she took it to his bed noticed that he was reading a book about Columbus and the discovery of America. In the afternoon he began to suffer acutely and called out to Frieda in his alarm that he was delirious. For highly imaginative men whose minds are constantly full of images, delirium must represent a special fear and danger. There is a reasonably detailed record of how, after a stroke, Henry James began to confuse memories with reality and yet he retained a dim awareness that he was often incoherent and perhaps ridiculous. Lawrence was by contrast able to retain full mental control until the very end ('Don't cry', he said sharply to Frieda when she observed his tortured face), so that what he meant when he said he was delirious is rather different. Like Pushkin, who when he was dying reported that he could see himself across the room, Lawrence complained specifically of being able to see his own body lying opposite him on a table. Because these relatively common out-of-body experiences are suggestive of that death Donne describes in which the soul leaves the body, they are frequently given a religious connotation by either those who experience them or the people to whom they are recounted. But in Lawrence they produced only terror and alarm and he asked the women who were near to hold on to him as if by doing so they could secure his now uncertain tenure on earth. Barby and Frieda therefore had to take turns in putting their arms round his shoulders although help was now on hand in the form of Aldous and, more particularly, Maria Huxley. They had not been at the Villa Robermond when he first arrived there because they had gone to see a friend, the poet Robert Nichols who was staying with his wife in Villefranche, just a little along the coast from Nice; but they arrived back in Vence on what was now a Sunday afternoon to do what they could in the crisis which had developed. Sensitive and highly strung, Maria had once attempted suicide in the days before she had met Huxley at Garsington. Now on this Sunday afternoon, although Aldous was all solicitude, it was Maria who held Lawrence's head between her two hands to soothe him in his anguished delirium, a gesture from which he seems to have derived a special comfort.

In the nineteenth-century accounts of 'the good death', the protagonists offer encouraging as well as final words to their entourage (as if the obligation to cheer its members up lay on them), and express total confidence in being about to depart to a better life. It is hard to find convincing, secular equivalents of the good Christian death. This is what Denys Arcand attempted to do in his film *The Barbarian Invasions* where the protagonist is able to gather round him in the house near the lake all his best and oldest friends who eat fine food, drink fine wine, and talk with the dying man about the old times. Something of the spirit Arcand is looking for may also be hinted at in the records of Chekhov's death. The spa in which he died was German but it was apparently a feature of both Russian and German medical etiquette that a doctor at the deathbed of a medical colleague, once he had decided there was no more hope, should indicate that fact by ordering a bottle of champagne. Chekhov's doctor did this and his gesture would seem to chime in with a common hope of secularists that, if once we knew that we had only a short time to live, we would make sure we made the most of it. If life is all there is and not that unsatisfactory transitional stage to an infinitely preferable way of being implicit in Christian belief, it needs to be lived out as fully as possible until the very end. This is the position evoked or perhaps also parodied in the joke about the man who has been forbidden to smoke but always carries an unlighted cigarette in his mouth on the grounds that, if he is ever told he had five minutes to live, he would not have to waste time looking for a packet.

Making the most of one's last days or hours is not as easy as the healthy sometimes make it sound. There must often have been a grimmer reality behind secular tales of final celebrations as it has now been established there often was behind the nineteenth-century Christian narratives of the good death. After all, how many condemned men have actually enjoyed the slap-up meal they have been allowed the night before their execution? In their case, the threats to healthy appetite are probably psychological but in the case of those in the situation of Denys Arcand's hero or of Chekhov, they are likely to be physiological also. The friends of the dying man in *The Barbarian Invasions* cook a splendid valedictory meal but sadly note that this is the first occasion on which he has refused fresh truffles and that he is not able to take even a sip of particularly remarkable wine. Because Chekov's tuberculosis had travelled to his digestive organs (as it probably had also to those of Lawrence), eating and drinking gave him almost as much trouble in his last years as breathing. In the state he was in when he died, he is unlikely to have enjoyed even the finest vintage of Veuve Cliquot. Lawrence was in a similar state and with breathing so difficult and painful that perhaps the only thing which could have temporarily prolonged his life was oxygen. But he had already tried that and decided it made him feel worse rather than better. For Frieda's sake, this was perhaps a good thing. In *The Magic Mountain*, Hans Castorp has been puzzled by strangely shaped bottles outside the doors of one or two of the rooms on his corridor in the sanatorium. He learns that they contain oxygen which can be used to prolong the life of the dying for a few extra hours. Each bottle costs 6 francs and he hears later that a young widow has been left penniless because her dying husband consumed so many of them. Walking with Hans along his corridor one day, the sanatorium's chief doctor, Hofrat Behrens, complains mildly about his '*moribundus*' in number 27. 'Five dozen flasks of oxygen he's had all together, yesterday and today', he says, 'the soak'. As Behrens then enters room 27, Hans hears him say, with the breezy medical efficiency which is very much his own: 'Well, my dear Reuter, what do you say—shall we crack open another bottle?' One can only hope, and indeed believe, that when Chekhov's doctor proposed champagne he employed a different tone.

Instead of oxygen, Lawrence called for morphine: 'I ought to have some morphine now' was Frieda's account of what he said while Barby remembered, 'I must have morphia'. His general attitude to pain-killing drugs, or to those like alcohol which work to lessen physical but chiefly psychological discomfort, was complicated; but he seems to have made relatively little use of either. This was not for any orthodox moral reasons. Lawrence followed his father in approving of alcohol and would make fun of the humourless way his mother told the story from the Temperance League about the young abstainer who was made to drink beer when wicked colleagues poured it down a gap in his front teeth. There is evidence that when he was in New Mexico he experimented with peyote, a hallucinatory drug common among the Indians. But in general he disliked having his senses dulled or his mind altered because he was happiest, or at least most content, when he could feel that the world with which he was engaged was real, even if it brought him pain. Perhaps because he had such a strong tendency to solipsism, he wanted above all to feel himself face to face with things as they really were. Mexico had satisfied him more than any other of the countries he had lived in because he felt that at least there one could be in contact with the natural and human world as it really was, so different from that lovey-dovey, love-thy-neighbour version which in Europe had been exposed as a sham by the horrors of the First World War. He did not want this real world to be obscured from him either by illusions concerning its nature, or by substances which allowed him to escape its grip. There is a remarkable moment in *Women in Love* when the slightly mad Mrs Crich contemplates her husband's dead body and says, 'Beautiful, beautiful as if life had never touched you—never touched you.—God send I look different.—I hope I shall look my years when I am dead,' and she then screams at the children, 'None of you look like this when you are dead.' Life has not marked Thomas Crich because he has found means of evading its realities. No one who looked closely at the photographic portraits taken of Lawrence in his last years, or at the Davidson bust, could have said the same of him, but by the time he asked Frieda and Barby to find some morphine he must have felt that he had been marked by life quite enough. His request was the equivalent of the one he and his sister Ada must have fervently believed their dying mother would have made, had she been in any state to do so. It is reasonable to conjecture that what he now needed, and was requesting, was someone with the decisiveness he and Ada had once shown, that he was speaking in a code which she above all would have understood.

The problem was the usual one of procurement. As a doctor Chekhov was able to take a stock of morphine with him to Germany but although Lawrence may have been able to bring from the hospital some of the codeine he had been taking, there was no morphine easily available. Barby set off to look for the Corsican doctor but it was Sunday and he was not at home. She therefore went to see the proprietor of the hotel where Frieda had stayed when she first came to Vence and persuaded him to ring the Ad Astra to ask whether Dr Madinier could come to the villa to administer the drug. Not surprisingly he at first refused. Lawrence had after all discharged himself and was no longer Madinier's responsibility. Marcus Paterson, the doctor in charge of the Frimley sanatorium in Surrey, was always very annoyed when patients discharged themselves and is reputed to have said to one man who insisted on leaving: 'Tell your widow to stay in touch with us. We need the details of your death for our records.' But the Frimley was a charitable institution, at the prison-camp end of the spectrum of sanatoria, and Paterson was a notorious disciplinarian. Madinier was eventually persuaded to come and, although he complained all the way in the taxi from the Ad Astra, Barby was relieved to see how impeccably he behaved once he saw Lawrence.

The morphine Madinier administered produced the desired if rather too long-delayed effect and Lawrence fell into a coma with Frieda holding on to one of his ankles. Maria stayed with her while Aldous and Barby again went to find the Corsican doctor in the expectation that more morphine would be needed later. But when they returned to the villa around 11 o'clock, after another unsuccessful search, Lawrence was already dead. He had died around 10 with Frieda still holding his ankle. As she movingly put it: 'he was breathing more peacefully, and then suddenly there were gaps in the breathing. The moment came when the thread of life tore in his heaving chest, his face changed, his cheeks and jaw sank, and death took hold of him.' This is closely observed. In the surviving casts of Keats's death mask there are still signs of the linen shroud which was used to tie up his sunken jaw while the mask was being made.

'And say shall I groan in dying | as I twist the sweaty sheet', writes John Betjeman in his 'Cottage Hospital', 'Or gasp for breath uncrying | as I feel my senses drowned'. James Elroy Flecker, who was born only one year before Lawrence but who died of tuberculosis in 1915, had similar apprehensions in his 'No coward's song':

> I am afraid to think about my death
> When it shall be, and whether in great pain
> I shall rise up and fight the air for breath
> Or calmly wait the bursting of my brain.

Lawrence was fortunate enough to die in a morphine-induced sleep or coma. He had fought fiercely against his illnesses but it may be that, at the very last, he had been able to help himself. Throughout his career, but especially during the period when he was writing *Women in Love* and his *Studies in Classic American Literature*, he had been preoccupied with the way certain people are able to use their will-power to disrupt the harmony of their relation to their environment and go against what might be called the natural processes of their living. One particularly striking illustration of this was the determination of certain individuals to cling to life beyond a point where it was reasonable to do so, as he increasingly felt had been his mother's case. There was then of course a difficult and subtle distinction to be made between this illegitimate use of the will-power and the courage required to live a full life and die gamely. In spite of all his years of fierce resistance and denial, it might just be that in dying when he did Lawrence showed that he knew how to make this distinction and when to relax his will. The suggestion can only ever be highly speculative but there might be some support for it in the reaction of his doctors. When Lawrence left the Ad Astra, Dr Madinier had thought him very sick but he nevertheless expressed surprise that he died so quickly. After learning of his death, Andrew Morland wrote to Koteliansky on 9 March, 'When I heard from the doctors at Vence that he was not responding to treatment I feared that there was little chance of recovery but I certainly had no expectations of the end coming so suddenly.' Lawrence had confounded some of his doctors by living much longer than they anticipated but he seems then to have confounded others by dying quicker than they thought he would.

$$\boxed{13}$$

Famous Last Words

When a great deal of attention is focused on the hour of death, everything associated with it becomes important. Donne's onlookers would not only be watching to see when the dying man stopped breathing but also listening to hear whatever requests, advice, or famous last words he might utter. The higher the social rank the more intense the listening was likely to be. Those who surrounded the deathbed of Elizabeth I, for example, were said to have waited anxiously for her to name James VI of Scotland as her successor and thereby give an added legitimacy to arrangements which had already been made. That she did in fact name him has been described as legend by one biographer who suggests that, by the time her councillors 'stood round her great bed' on 23 March 1603 (the day before she died), Elizabeth had lost the power of speech. Yet if she did manage to utter something it would have been regarded as highly significant while, at lower social levels, the mystery and awe surrounding death always tended to confer a special if less specific authority on the last things said.

In December 1603, sometime during the night before he was due to be executed, and after James had been on the English throne for only nine months, Sir Walter Raleigh wrote a magnificent letter to his wife, 'my last words in these my last

---

---

lines' as he put it. He urged her not to be too downcast ('your mourning cannot avail me that am but dust'), described the state of his financial affairs, warned her against future suitors while at the same time insisting that she should remarry, and concluded by saying that his letter was written with 'the dying hand of sometime thy husband, but now (alas!) overthrown'. The mixture in this document of warm affection with thoughtfulness, and of pragmatism with religious feeling, means that it easily survives the inconvenient fact that Raleigh was reprieved at the last minute and not executed in December 1603 but all of fifteen years later. The case of Chidiock Tichbourne is instructively different. He was a young man condemned to be hung, drawn, and quartered because of his involvement in a Catholic plot relatively early in Elizabeth's reign and he left behind a short elegy of three stanzas. This poem was later much anthologized, not because it has any unusual literary merit—it is in fact rather banal—but because its subtitle reads 'written with his own hand on the eve of his execution'. Had Tichbourne been reprieved as Raleigh was, it is very doubtful whether anyone would have ever heard of it.

Last words take many forms, from elaborate written addresses to 'Citizen' Kane's single enigmatic muttered word 'Rosebud', the trigger for the investigation of his character in the famous film which bears his name. What certainly still pleases is when the final words to be recorded—or invented—seem eminently characteristic because then the sting of death is partly drawn, and the dead can be thought of as having continued to be 'themselves' until the very end. It would be disappointing to learn that Heinrich Heine did not claim that he knew his sins would be forgiven because forgiveness was part of God's job description (*c'est son métier*); or that Oscar Wilde, contemplating the vulgar wallpaper of the Paris hotel room where he lay dying, did not insist that either he or it would have to go. In a more recent example, it seems fitting that the rumbustious Irish playwright Brendan Behan should have blessed the nun who was tending him, and hoped that all her sons might become bishops. All these well-known cases require a certain latitude in the interpretation of 'last'. After a stroke preliminary to the one which finally killed him, Henry James told a friend that he had heard a voice saying distinctly, 'So here it is at last, the distinguished thing.' These cannot have been literally James's last words but they are so eminently 'Jamesian' that it seems appropriate to regard them in that light.

The obvious problem is that, in the very last moments of life, pain, delirium, or the effect of drugs are always likely to prevent the dying from uttering words which are worthwhile, or even intelligible (which is why execution often provides the most favourable occasions for them). Anyone anxious that their own last words should make a good impression, and who does not expect to be executed, would therefore do well to rehearse. Alien as the anxiety to make a good impression was to the later Lawrence, this is what he could be said to have done when, early in 1925, he was lying gravely ill in Oaxaca. Here was another moment in his life when he 'nearly died' but one when Frieda recalled that, for the first time since she had known him, he appeared momentarily to give up hope. This is the special circumstance which gives to what he apparently then told her the authority of last words rehearsed, or held in reserve. 'If I die', she reports Lawrence as saying, '*nothing has mattered but you, nothing at all.*'

Certain words can be too easily consecrated as the last because they are so gratifying to the recipients. There was no one in Oaxaca who could have confirmed Frieda's testimony but that her husband should have felt that all his other relationships had been as nothing compared to the one he had enjoyed with her accords well enough with what we know of his life. It marks as authentic what he is reported as saying: the kind of pondered, final remark of a man who feels that if he does not express what is on his mind immediately, he might not be able to do so later. As Frieda was fond of telling her husband, and anyone else who would listen, he was in a poor emotional state when in 1912 she first met him. Successive close relationships with two loving, intelligent teachers from his local area had broken down, with lasting damage to both women, and Lawrence was still haunted by memories of his mother, who had died more than a year before. Frieda's relaxed attitude to sex, her cosmopolitanism, and her combative temperament permanently altered the way he both lived and wrote. Since after his marriage Lawrence never settled long enough in one place to form lasting social ties, and as a writer never had to 'go out to work', he and Frieda lived together more closely than most couples do. They could both reach points where they found the resulting intimacy intolerable, but their periodic separations always ended in Frieda being able to demonstrate that his need was greater than hers. As Huxley later put it in a letter, 'he felt towards her as a man might feel towards his own liver: the liver may give trouble from time to time, but it remains one of the vital organs, absolutely necessary to survival.' Other friends of

Lawrence were more insistent in suggesting she was bad for him, in part because their famous quarrels drove him to a pitch of exasperation dangerous for someone whose health was so fragile, and also because she did not seem to notice how fragile it in fact was. Yet all of them had to concede that he would never leave her. Those who in the later years were able to observe how agitated Lawrence became when Frieda was a few hours late returning from one of her combined visits to her family and Angelo Ravagli might well feel that, although she had liberated him from bondage to his mother, it was only at the expense of exchanging one dependence for another; but they were aware that he could not do without her. They knew that she mattered supremely, as Frieda was happy to report her husband had acknowledged in Oaxaca.

Lawrence did not die in Oaxaca in 1925 but in Vence in 1930. If his last words then had included some kind of repetition of what he had said in Mexico, Frieda would no doubt have been the first to say so; but the only memorable direct reference to her by the dying Lawrence was recorded by Robert Nichols. He was told by Aldous Huxley that on the Thursday or Friday before his death on the Sunday Lawrence had said, '*Frieda, you have killed me.*' These are very different last words from those Lawrence had pronounced in Oaxaca but not necessarily in contradiction with them, although quite what they mean is not easy to determine. Huxley himself would no doubt have recalled the occasion in Paris when the return of Frieda was instrumental in making Lawrence cancel the appointment he had made to have an X-ray. Others might have conjectured that knowledge of his wife's affair with Angelo Ravagli had drained away some of the energy and will which Lawrence needed to fight his disease. But perhaps the words alluded more generally to the extraordinary turbulence of his relationship with Frieda in the early years.

One of the many original features of Lawrence's fourth novel, *The Rainbow*, is the depiction of the early married life of Will and Anna Brangwen and the extraordinarily violent oscillations between love and hate which they both have to endure. That the passionate intensity of their relationship is largely autobiographical is confirmed by Lawrence's record of similar oscillations in the poems he wrote during his first few years with Frieda. Other people the couple knew were able to become aware of this intensity when they saw blows exchanged and the occasional item of crockery flying across the room. There was also a good deal of verbal aggression which neither party bothered to conceal. Lawrence, for example, always disliked Frieda smoking. This may have been because he himself had been warned off cigarettes by various doctors but was much more probably a consequence of his upbringing. In his mother's time any women seen smoking in public risked being regarded as a prostitute, or at least someone of loose morals. Especially aggravating to him was the way Frieda would let a lighted cigarette dangle from the corner of her wide, expressive gunslinger's mouth while she half-closed her eyes against the smoke. Once in Taos while she was doing this he burst out with, 'Take that dirty cigarette out of your mouth! And stop sticking out that fat belly of yours!' While the rest of the company looked on appalled Frieda replied, 'You'd better stop that talk or I'll tell about *your* things.' Exchanges such as this were so frequent that Lawrence's 'You have killed me' may not have shocked Frieda unduly. His words could have signalled his recognition that so much intensity in the past, so relatively little quiet domestic bliss, had taken its toll although if they did, and were meant as a reproach, they were both unfair and uncharacteristic. Conflict was meat and drink to Lawrence and essential to his creativity. Had he been forced to make the choice, he would certainly have opted to die early from the stress of his marriage rather than late from the boredom of a quiet life. In his own psychosomatic view of illness, moreover, including his mother's cancer, it was not only stress itself which was the causative agent but also strict self-control, the repression of angry and hostile feelings. Although the decision he clearly made after meeting Frieda to live spontaneously and never hold back led to stormy scenes, they would therefore have been seen by him not so much as a cause of disease, but rather as a prophylactic against it.

Lawrence's claim that Frieda had killed him is very hard to interpret and much depends on what is now irrecoverable: the way his words were pronounced. It is possible, although not perhaps very likely, that the tone was one of semi-humorous exasperation at the ineptitude of Frieda's nursing. He had complained in the past that she had the heavy hands of a German soldier and, although he clearly preferred her ministrations to those of the hired nurse, there were others who were with him at the end from whom he derived more comfort. It was during these last hours or days, for example, that Lawrence said that Maria Huxley had hands like his mother. This helps to explain why, in those moments of extreme distress and panic before Dr Madinier arrived with his morphine injection, he felt so much relief when Maria held his head. The two of them were clearly left alone from time to time and at one point Lawrence seized both her wrists and cried out: '*Maria, Maria, don't let me die.*' These were the most salient of Lawrence's final words which Maria Huxley remembered and they have poignancy absent from the other candidates on offer.

It seems appropriate that Lawrence's various last words should have been addressed to women since women, or his relations with them, played such a crucial role in his life. His first relationship had been with Jessie Chambers, whom he would see every Sunday at the Congregationalist chapel in Eastwood, and visit at the nearby farm her father rented. In those days Jessie was the only person to whom he would show everything he wrote and she was consequently crucial to his development. It would be no exaggeration to say that she worshipped him and she was certainly anxious to minister to his every need. When he pressed her to have sex with him, without any very firm expectation of marriage, her agreement represented a momentous decision for someone of her period, background, and religious beliefs. Although Lawrence rejected Christianity relatively early in his life, he would later suggest that the only form of it which he found at all acceptable was Roman Catholicism. The last rites for the dying in Catholicism are commonly preceded by confession and, if Lawrence had chosen that route, at the top of his list of sins to confess might well have been his treatment of Jessie Chambers. She dealt with her abandonment, and with the remarkably frank and hurtful way Lawrence represented their relationship in *Sons and Lovers*, by cutting off all communications. Yet he was never very far from her thoughts. She records that on Sunday 2 March 1930 she heard a voice saying, as distinctly as if Lawrence were there in the same room with her in England: '*Can you remember only the pain and none of the joy?*' These were his last words to Jessie who claimed that it was only on the following day that she had learnt of his death.

There are two kinds of last words. One consists of those remembered as such by particular individuals, as Jessie and Maria remembered theirs, and the other, the actual last words spoken. Frieda recalled that after being given the morphine, and before dropping into a coma, Lawrence had said, '*I am better now.*' But another version comes from Ida Hughes-Stanton. She was the wife of the man who had carried Lawrence into the Ad Astra and claimed to have heard from him, almost certainly via Barby, that Lawrence's positively final remark had been '*Wind my watch*'. Neither of these two phrases seems especially memorable or significant but then, to the other burdens of dying, why should the extra one be added of saying (or writing) something impressive? It seems hard that writers in particular, men and women who have produced in their lives hundreds of thousands of memorable words, should be expected to utter at the very last, one or two of special resonance and significance. It is partly a question of how far our social obligations should extend. The nineteenth-century Spanish general who declared during his final confession that he did not have to forgive his enemies because he had had them all shot seems to have been protesting against that 'performance aspect' of dying which has largely disappeared along with the Christian beliefs which helped to sustain it. Against Addison's request that his nephew should be called so that he could see how a Christian might die could be placed the angry response which has been attributed to the dying Karl Marx. 'Go on, get out,' he apparently said to his housekeeper, 'Last words are for fools who haven't said enough!'

Even angrier is a passage from Henri de Montherlant's *Mors et Vita* which appears as the epigraph to the harrowing narrative of tuberculosis and suffering in Derek Lindsay's *The Rack*:

> All those people who utter famous last words as they are dying, who stiffen into attitudes as if the stiffening which will finally come in three days were not enough, people who in three days will no longer exist and yet still want to be admired, who pose and lie with their last breath as if to say: see how I can die, these are called heroes. For me they are miserable creatures. If I want to cry out, must I stifle my cry to please the onlookers and make them admire me! I would rather make my cry louder so as to show for one last time how little I care about the world and the world's opinion.

This is impressive but possibly too vehement and it could be said that anyone so concerned to defy the opinion of the world, even on his deathbed, must still be in its thrall. Since Lawrence died so relatively quietly and privately a more suitable comment on the convention of last words can perhaps be found in the mild irony of one of his biographers, Hugh Kingsmill. 'My one regret', Kingsmill is reported to have said as he was dying, 'is that I have used too many commas. On the question of semi-colons, I have nothing to reproach myself.'

14

Funeral

After Lawrence's death, Frieda remembered the shape of his feet in the slippers which lay neatly under his bed and she was struck by a face from which all suffering had been wiped. It was, she said, 'as if I had never known him or seen him in all the completeness of his being'. There may be an echo here of one of Lawrence's earliest and most successful short stories, 'Odour of Chrysanthemums', towards the end of which a dead miner is being laid out by his mother and his young wife. For the mother he has reverted to the child and young man she once knew so well, but the wife is overcome with a sense that in death her husband has become alien, a stranger.

Lawrence was often preoccupied with how people look just after they have died, principally because he nursed his own mother in her last days. He wrote several poems in which he described her appearance after death as that of a virgin, 'like a maiden dreaming' as he put it in one of his letters; and he suggested that it had returned her to girlhood. Implicit in that suggestion was the curious and unhealthy notion that his mother was more truly his own after her death because she was then free from contamination of any contact with his father. Frieda did not like these poems and there is a hint in his portrayal of Mrs Crich's response to the death of her husband in *Women in Love* that Lawrence came not to like them either. One of the last short stories he wrote was called 'The Lovely Lady' and concerns the death of a remarkably well-preserved but selfish old woman. When her son comes to view the corpse, she is described as 'pretty again, but shrunken, like a little old child', and it is said that what her face expresses is 'the pathos of a maid who has died virgin and unlived . . . hardened to her own will'. This reads like a harsh reversal of judgement by Lawrence on the mother who had once meant so much to him. If his own face after death was indeed wiped free of suffering, and other consequences of interaction with the world, all Frieda may have been recording was a common physiological phenomenon: many people report that the faces of the recently dead can have a serenity which makes them seem more youthful. But if in describing it what she said contains a faint reminder of the young miner's wife in 'Odour of Chrysanthemums', then the appropriate response might be similar to the one Lawrence himself once gave when she was riding with him in New Mexico and exclaimed how wonderful it was to feel her horse's movements between her thighs. 'Rubbish, Frieda', he had then snapped, 'don't talk like that. You have been reading my books.'

The local by-laws dictated that Lawrence's body should be quickly disposed of and his burial was therefore arranged for 4 p.m. on 4 March, the Tuesday following his death (Frieda may have considered cremation but there were no facilities at hand). For the manner of the burial she was faced by what is now a very familiar dilemma for those who do not belong to a particular religious community: what kind of ceremony or ritual there should be. Like so many other towns in an area which had for many years been colonized by the English, there was in Vence an

English church. In such a small community the resident vicar or chaplain must quickly have heard of Lawrence's death and he offered to come to the funeral and say a few prayers. It seems right that Frieda should have refused this offer when one thinks of the number of unsympathetic portraits of Anglican clergy there are in her husband's work. Brought up as a non-conformist, Lawrence had an especially sharp awareness of the falsities Anglicans can be led into by the close association of their church with the middle and upper, but not the lower, urban classes of English society. And then, more obviously, although Lawrence was (as he often protested) a religious man, he was certainly not a Christian when he died.

The speed with which the funeral was arranged necessarily limited the number of people able to attend. Apart from Frieda, Barby, the Huxleys, and Ida Rauh, the di Chiaras may have been present and Achsah Brewster certainly came over from Bandol. Lawrence's Paris publisher, Edward Titus, arrived, to pay tribute to the dead but also because he had to be in the South of France to meet his wife, who had sailed directly to Cannes from New York. He was in addition keen to settle some on-going business matters with Frieda, who, without her husband's knowledge, had begun to take control of his publishing affairs a month before his death. This had made Titus nervous but when he had written to ask whether Lawrence would mind, Frieda had blithely replied, 'Yes, Lawr would mind my writing to you about business, but I don't think very profoundly and he hates it so himself anyhow.'

Previously alerted to Lawrence's state by Huxley, Robert Nichols also drove over from Villefranche with his wife for the funeral. A poet who had some popular success in the early months of the war, Nichols had been invalided out of the army with shell shock in 1915. After a long convalescence he had pursued a career as poet, novelist, and dramatist (a play of his from 1928 was a success in New York), and travelled widely. He was above all a close friend of Huxley but Nichols had met Lawrence during the war and saw him again in 1929 when they happened to be in Majorca at the same time. They never got on especially well and Nichols was later to complain of a certain element of impatience and condescension in Lawrence's attitude towards him and his lack of scruple about 'wading into one's inner sanctum and denouncing the furniture and throwing it about'. It was largely therefore to support the Huxleys that he had come to Vence yet, as he made clear in the long and detailed account of the funeral he wrote to Henry Head (the distinguished neurologist who had treated him for shell shock), he also wanted to pay tribute to someone he regarded as a great writer and, for all his faults, a great man.

Nichols and his wife arrived before lunch at the Villa Robermond and he describes well the tension during the long wait until 4 o'clock. When Barby opened the door of the bedroom to take in the flowers which were now frequently arriving, he could see Lawrence's feet covered by a sheet but also, beyond the feet, his 'little Greek satyr's beard sticking up'. Every time Barby came out of the room she was crying. What particularly struck him was the contrast between the relative calm of the large and voluble Frieda, who nevertheless occasionally fell silent and stared in an odd manner, and the devastation written all over the pale but now greyish face of the slightly built Maria Huxley. From time to time, he says, Maria shivered and enormous tears gathered in her light blue, red-lidded eyes. Despite her condition, it was she who was busy when Nichols arrived, scrubbing out the villa's kitchen and trying to rectify the 'hell of an unwholesome mess' Frieda had already managed to make there. Aldous meanwhile was frustrated that Frieda seemed unwilling to take even the most ordinary precautions 'such as burning clothes etc.', but if this was in fact the burden of Huxley's complaint he was less scientifically up to the mark than we always think of him as being, and a good deal more superstitious. When Keats was dying in Rome he asked to be moved into a room next to the one he occupied because it was bigger. Severn was obliged to effect the removal without the knowledge of the landlady because the bigger room contained valuable items of furniture and it was the rule in Rome that all the contents of a room in which a consumptive had died should be burned. Since tuberculosis is infectious but not contagious, it is highly improbable that this did any good, or that burning Lawrence's clothes would have made the slightest difference. Nor could it have had much effect that, after his death, the villa in which he had died was fumigated in accordance with local regulations.

The hearse which came to carry the coffin to the cemetery was drawn by a single horse. While Nichols's own car was used for others of those present he, the Huxleys, and Frieda were crammed into a small taxi which had to follow the hearse at a snail's pace across town (the cemetery was close to the Ad Astra). This is the way things were done, and are still often done but, as Nichols says, there is something in it of 'going to an execution'. The hope is presumably that members of a community have an opportunity to pay their respects to one of their number who has died, and to the fact of Death itself. But now that the idea of community has been so much complicated, and the hearse with its following cars often has to take a motorway to reach its destination, that hope is rarely fulfilled. Nichols was, however, gratified that, apart from one reluctant Englishman whom he was obliged to stare out of countenance, all those who saw the hearse took off their hats or crossed themselves: 'These Southerners respect death,' he noted and their gestures helped to assuage the obscure feeling he had that the passing of such a great writer should somehow be more marked. Frieda was gratified by the gestures of the locals as well, but also by the fact that the sun had come out and it was a fine March day. This is how he would have liked it, she told Nichols, and then, in a reference to the funeral party, 'just friends'. There would in the future be many more of these confident interpretations of what her dead husband's thoughts and feelings would have been.

Waiting at the cemetery to join the others was someone who was like Nichols in also feeling that the occasion was too low-key. This was the painter Frank Budgen, who happened to be in Vence in order to provide support for his friend Louis Sargent. The chest complaint from which Sargent suffered remains unspecified, but he was being treated by the same Dr Maestracci whom Frieda had engaged when Lawrence left the Ad Astra and it was from him that he and Budgen learned of Lawrence's death. They immediately sent flowers to the Villa Robermond with a note to explain that, although they did not know Lawrence personally, they greatly admired his work (according to Nichols, the flowers were red carnations and Frieda was much touched); and they also decided to attend the funeral. In a letter he wrote describing the proceedings, Budgen says how surprised he was to find so few people there given all the 'writers and painters, English and American, who live here and at St Paul and Cagnes and all around this part of the world'. Although he does not say so, one notable absentee was Wells, who was perhaps not anxious to have to accept the most effective refutation any sick person can ever offer to the kind of diagnosis he had proposed. Although Budgen painted, he is best remembered today for his memoir of James Joyce, one of his closest friends. Looking back, it seems as if at the beginning of 1930 Joyce and Lawrence were the two greatest, non-American writers in English, with the possible addition of Virginia Woolf; but they did not appreciate one another. When he was writing his Australian novel *Kangaroo* in 1922, Lawrence had been intrigued by rumours of Joyce's *Ulysses*: here was perhaps a novelist after his own heart, breaking bounds, challenging literary convention, and attracting censorship. But once he was able to read the novel, he was very disappointed and inclined to feel that parts of it were pornographic. His friends the Crosbys were keen Joyceans and insisted on playing him a record of Joyce reading the Aeolus episode from *Ulysses* to which Lawrence's response was 'Yes, I thought so, a preacher, a Jesuit preacher who believes in the cross upside down'. The preacher concerned was no more complimentary, meeting a suggestion made in 1929 that Lawrence should be asked to contribute to a proposed new journal with, 'That man really writes very badly. You might ask for something from his friend Aldous Huxley, who at least dresses decently.' The hostility between Joyce and Lawrence, who probably never met, may have encouraged the feeling which developed later that it is possible to admire either one or the other, but not both; yet the presence of a committed Joycean like Budgen at Lawrence's funeral suggests that, in 1930, this was not yet the case.

Budgen and Sargent came to the funeral with their wives, one of whom counted the participants and calculated that, including themselves but not the undertaker and his assistants, the number was twenty-two. This leaves several people to be accounted for but the hired nurse may have attended and, during her short time in Vence, Frieda seems already to have formed one or two friendships among the locals. Apart from feeling that more people should have been there, Budgen wondered whether four of Lawrence's friends might not have carried the coffin to the grave instead of the assistants, and he also thought that one of those friends, Huxley perhaps, could have said a few words. The advantage of this was that it would at least have slowed down 'the tempo of the proceedings'. As he rightly says, however, if one rejects the current forms of burial, it is no easy job to invent new ones. According to Nichols, after the assistants had lowered the coffin into the grave, they paused as if expecting a speech but instead Frieda came forward and dropped a flower on top of it. Most of her party then did the same and they also followed her example after she had taken over from the undertakers the task of arranging various wreaths around the grave, once it had been filled. The exception was Maria who was weeping and paralysed with grief. Frieda was content that her husband was being buried in such a beautiful spot, in a plot of land which slopes away from the town and which at that date allowed fine views across an uncluttered valley of orange groves with glimpses of the Mediterranean in the distance. But Maria was preoccupied with the loss of someone she had known at least as long as she had known her husband, and of whom she had been very fond.

The extent or depth of grief is very difficult to judge. One of Lawrence's early poems begins with 'My love lies underground | With her face upturned to mine, | And her mouth unclosed in a last long kiss | That ended her life and mine'. The reference is to his mother and the poem goes on to describe the speaker's casual, brief flirtation or affair with a country girl in spite of his 'stream of life' being 'deathward set'. It ends:

> Grief, grief, I suppose and sufficient
> Grief makes us free
> To be faithless and faithful together
> As we have to be.

This difficult formula of being 'faithless and faithful together' points towards the recognition that dead loved ones are necessarily betrayed by all those who want to go on living (as Dora Carrington must have felt when she committed suicide rather than live on after the death of Lytton Strachey). Because the dead loved one lying underground is Lawrence's mother, one could say that he found articulation of the formula easier than its emotional acceptance. It is no necessary criticism of Frieda to note that in her case intellectual and emotional acceptance were much more at one, and that she was not likely to be a victim of what some psychologists have termed 'disordered mourning'. When Robert Nichols arrived in Vence and witnessed the distress of Maria Huxley—'little Maria' as he calls her—his first, instinctive thought was that she was 'far worthier of Lawrence than Frieda'. But grief is not a competition and its outward manifestations are hard to read.

Both Lawrence and Huxley were convinced that the very public and demonstrative manner in which Middleton Murry expressed his grief after the death of Katherine Mansfield was factitious. In *Point Counter Point* there is an obvious portrait of Murry as Burlap, someone who by 'a process of intense concentration on the idea of his loss and grief' has succeeded in churning up within himself agonies which are in no way proportionate or even related to the feeling he had for his wife while she was alive. 'At the end of a few days of spiritual masturbation', Huxley writes, Burlap was rewarded with 'a mystical realization of his own unique and incomparable piteousness'. At the heart of this description is the charge that, in his mourning for Mansfield, Murry was far more concerned with himself than with her. That was almost certainly true yet it is rare that grief is entirely disinterested. Maria Huxley might well have said that she grieved at the loss in Lawrence of such a dear and close friend but the unavoidable self-interest of this natural feeling is brought out by Dr Johnson when he begins an elegy on the death of one of his own friends with,

> Condemn'd to hope's delusive mine,
> As on we toil from day to day,
> By sudden blasts, and slow decline,
> Our social comforts drop away.

Many of Lawrence's friends would have felt his death as the deprivation of a 'social comfort' while the more vulnerable among them would also have taken it as a reminder of their own mortality and mourned in their grief the sadness of the human condition. Although Frieda might have shared this first feeling if not the second, her situation as the widow was complicated and very different from Maria's. As the person who had nursed Lawrence more than any other, her disinterested thankfulness that his sufferings were over must have been mixed with some relief at no longer being responsible for trying to alleviate them; and her sorrow at the death of someone who was still only middle-aged, and might therefore have had many more years before him, must also have been accompanied by some pity for herself as the one bereft. In any relationship there is usually one partner more dependent than the other. Although Lawrence was far more emotionally dependent on Frieda than she was on him, in practical matters the situation was reversed. He not only assumed the traditionally female roles of cooking and cleaning, in addition to mending the fuses and repairing the roof, but was 'the man of the house' insofar as he insisted on making all the financial or business arrangements. Commenting much later on Frieda's state after her husband's death Huxley wrote: 'One of the most curious facts about Frieda was her extreme helplessness when left alone to cope with a practical situation. . . . She had relied *totally* on Lawrence, and felt completely lost until she had found another man to support her.' It was this lostness for which she must in part have grieved but never to the extent of seeing herself, like Burlap, as an object of 'unique and incomparable piteousness'. Maria and Frieda were women in very different situations, and of very different temperaments, but they grieved as people usually do and without a hint of what, in his analysis of Murry, Huxley cruelly but not unfairly calls his 'spiritual masturbation'.

15

Pilgrims

The rapidity with which Lawrence was buried meant that there was no opportunity for members of his family, or for his friends from England, to attend the funeral. This particularly distressed his younger sister Ada, who had nursed her brother through several serious illnesses, lent him money during the war, and was the family member best equipped, through educational training and intelligence, to understand and follow his literary career. The letter Lawrence wrote from the Ad Astra to postpone the trips to France which Ada and Emily had planned for the end of February had made a special point of assuring them both that he was in no immediate danger. Now that he was dead they both of them, but Ada in particular, felt cheated of the opportunity of seeing him for one last time.

By the time Ada was able to get to Vence it is likely that Frieda had already had installed a headstone on what was previously the bare patch of ground under which Lawrence's body lay. How best to commemorate the dead was a subject which had much preoccupied him three years earlier when he had visited the Etruscan tombs in Tarquinia, Volterra, and other north Italian towns with Earl Brewster. In one of the best of his later books (*Etruscan Places*), he recorded the delight he had felt at the way the Etruscans treated death as a continuation of life, covering the walls of the underground tombs in which they buried their dead with wonderfully fresh images of eating, drinking, and outdoor enjoyment. He was struck by the absence from the frescos of gloomy notions of suffering or punishment and approved of what he took to be an Etruscan conception of the after-life as much like this one, only better. Frieda was in no position to provide Lawrence with a painted underground tomb but what she did instead was commission two local artisans to fix on a headstone a mosaic of his favourite symbol of a phoenix rising once again from the flames. Rough as this work was, it provided a focus for the many visitors who soon began to arrive, wanting to see the grave of the author whose works they admired so much. Much later, the house where he was born would also become an object of literary pilgrimage. To visit a birthplace can be informative because it allows for comparison between a person's origins and what they later achieved. Visiting a grave yields no information of that kind and is more obviously therefore an appropriate pretext for reflection and an overt means for demonstrating love and respect. Certainly it was to demonstrate her own love that Ada took the long trip to the South of France and laid plants from her own, English garden on her brother's foreign grave.

As deeply affected as anyone from Eastwood by news of Lawrence's death was Jessie Chambers but whether what she experienced was the uncomplicated grief of Ada is doubtful. In two letters she wrote to her sister, one a week after hearing the news and the other in July, she omits to mention her vision but does insist that the Lawrence she knew was a 'living manifestation of God'. Pity and guilt are the feelings Jessie expresses in order to mask those of self-vindication, or even of a quietly triumphant satisfaction, which seem to have accompanied her distress. The guilt arose because when in 1913 Lawrence had sent her the proofs of *Sons and Lovers* and an accompanying letter in which he rather casually excused himself for the version of their relationship they contained, Jessie had returned the letter in her determination to make a clean break. Now when she remembered how he used to tell her, 'almost in despair', that as an artist he could do nothing without her, she wondered if she had done wrong. Was it then Lawrence who abandoned Jessie, uninformed readers of these phrases in one of her letters might ask, or she who had abandoned him? She could entertain this second possibility because, in her view, Lawrence made 'no development' after their parting: 'I think he has been afraid to face the real problems of his own personality, but I am sure he has suffered terribly, and endured awful loneliness.' Lawrence may have been 'deeply mistaken about life, poor chap', but when there was all the fuss with the authorities over his paintings and poems Jessie had felt like writing to him to assure him of her old affection. Since his death she has seen the letter which in November 1928 he had written to her brother David, not mentioning her but expressing warm, nostalgic feelings for his visits to her father's farm. This, and a few late writings of an autobiographical nature, have made her feel that, had Lawrence been able to live on 'we might have witnessed something in the nature of a miracle'. By a miracle she seems to have meant the return to his former and, in her view, real self of the man who had once meant everything to her.

It was sometimes said that Lawrence's relationship with Jessie broke down because she was too much like his mother. This seems strange at first since all the evidence we have suggests that Mrs Lawrence was a brisk, alert woman whereas Jessie was distinctly soulful, given to outbursts of feeling over a baby or a bunch of flowers which were so intense that they disconcerted members of the Lawrence family and made them dislike her. But one way in which the two women were similar is that they were both convinced that they understood Lawrence better than he understood himself, and that they knew what was best for him. ' "I can read him like a book", said my first lover of me', he once wrote, in an obvious reference to Jessie, and then added sarcastically, 'The book is in several volumes, dear'. However many volumes there were, Jessie's letters showed that once he was dead there was no way he could avoid her enveloping understanding and condescension. Characteristic of her habitual attitude had been her response when, two weeks before his mother's death, Lawrence rather timidly told her that he had become engaged to a friend of theirs who was also a teacher, Louie Burrows. With what she felt was her deep knowledge of his nature, Jessie told him that he was wrong to involve Louie in their own affairs, in the impasse of their relationship, implicitly suggesting that he was no more capable of breaking loose from her and making a free, rational choice than he was of escaping the influence of his mother.

There is a faint possibility that Jessie Chambers made the journey to Vence to visit Lawrence's grave, but Louie Burrows certainly did. She had been engaged to him for over a year but their relations became soured by her resolute determination to do nothing about the sexual frustration he frequently expressed, and by his apparent inability to save the hundred or so pounds they both had decided they needed before they could marry. When illness forced him to leave the teaching profession in 1912, he took the opportunity to ask her to release him from their engagement. She was very reluctant to do this and felt a sense of abandonment similar to Jessie's. In *Sons and Lovers* Lawrence describes how the young Paul Morel accidentally breaks the doll of his younger sister and deals with the discomfort he then experiences by ceremoniously cremating its remains in the back garden. It is an episode which suggests how intolerant Lawrence was of guilt feelings yet there is plenty in his life to indicate that he continued to feel uneasy about the way he had treated both Jessie and Louie. By returning his last letter, Jessie made things much easier for him but it is to Louie that he wrote his only recorded statement of frank apology. She does not seem to have replied and, as in 1930 she stood over what in a letter to Ada she described as the grave of the 'the poor lad' (echoing Jessie's 'poor chap'), her motives must have been mixed. In her life and Jessie's Lawrence had been a remarkable presence, investing the most ordinary, everyday matters with the acuteness and vitality of his observation, mimicking to comic perfection people they knew, widening their intellectual horizons with his enthusiasm for some new book, painter, or author and, latterly, bringing them exciting news of London literary life. There was nobody in their environment at all like him, which may be why Jessie was tempted to think him a manifestation of God. And yet he had left and, one might even say, betrayed them both. When Louie went to Vence, alone and without making any contact with Frieda, her posture may have been that of conventional mourning, and genuine grief almost certainly played an important part in her response; but had she been less well brought up, she might have been able to admit to herself that an additional reason for travelling so far was to drive a metaphorical stake through her former fiancé's heart.

This may seem exaggerated, especially as there are no surviving letters from Louie Burrows which indicate directly what her feelings were. An indirect indication of them is, however, apparent in the note she wrote to H. G. Wells in January 1933 about his recently published novel *The Bulpington of Blup*. If there were a prize for the novel in English with the worst title, *The Bulpington of Blup* might well win it, but it is in fact an impressive work which could have made Lawrence feel that Wells was back to something like his old form, had he lived long enough to read it. The protagonist of the novel is Theodore Bulpington, brought up in the genteel seaside resort of Blayport (which as a boy he conjectures was once called Blup). His parents are well-to-do former members of London's artistic community (his father had once contributed to *The Yellow Book*), and the emphasis in their household is on the importance of imagination. Partly as a result, Theodore grows up even more prone than most adolescents are to self-aggrandizing fantasies; he is *the* Bulpington of Blup. The only check to these wild imaginings comes from his friendship with Teddy and Margaret Broxted, the children of an eminent biologist who also lives in Blayport. Although they are much more down-to-earth, practical, and in touch with reality than he is, Theodore becomes warmly attached to them both and then falls in love with Margaret.

The crisis in the novel comes with the First World War. Both the Broxted children refuse to participate in the prevailing jingoistic mood and Teddy is eventually imprisoned as a conscientious objector; but Theodore's head is full of fantasies of himself as a military hero. These do not make him any the less tardy in enlisting. After he has finally done so, he uses the occasion to persuade Margaret to sleep with him. His first violent encounter in the war zone provokes a minor nervous collapse and he is transferred to an office job. When he has to go to the front line again and experience for the first time the realities of trench warfare, he runs away, passes out, and wakes up in the hands of a doctor who has to decide whether to classify him as a deserter, and thereby have him shot, or diagnose him as suffering from shell shock. Since he makes the humane choice, Theodore is allowed to return to England where, after his hospitalization, he begins to invent self-flattering narratives to explain his recent history and attempts to renew his sexual relationship with Margaret Broxted. But she is training to be a doctor, interested only in friendship and in any case about to marry someone else. Theodore nevertheless pesters her with letters so full of cringing appeals for sympathy, wild threats, and moral blackmail that they provoke a visit from her fiancé who turns out to be the same doctor who had saved Theodore's life by refusing to classify him as a deserter. After this shock he retires to a Devonshire cottage he has inherited and is last seen being lavishly wined and dined by two old ladies to whom he tells outrageously mendacious tales of his many heroic exploits during the war.

In her letter to Wells, Louie Burrows told him that she had been enthralled by the artistry and humour of *The Bulpington of Blup*, quite apart from the 'keen personal interest' it had aroused. She explained this personal interest by taking it for granted that the relationship between Theodore and Margaret had been deliberately based on that between herself and Lawrence and was so sure this was the case that she did not even bother to ask Wells for confirmation. 'In my heart I know that it was best you should have stripped Lawrence of his affectations and extravagance,' she wrote, 'They hid the core of him, which was good and fine'; and she went to say that she was 'very grateful and pleased that you have been so kind to Margaret'. As my lengthy plot summary of Wells's novel is meant to suggest, what is first of all remarkable in the startling assumptions of an otherwise sensible and intelligent woman which these words reveal is that Theodore, with his privileged background, war experience, and inability to tell the truth, is not even remotely like Lawrence (many of those in the literary world believed that the character was in fact based on Ford Madox Ford who was notorious for his fantasizing and had been in the army). But the second remarkable feature of Louie's mistake is that, by the end of his story, Theodore Bulpington has become so odious and contemptible that it ought to have been impossible to identity with him any person one had vaguely liked, let alone loved. The treatment is quite subtle, the degeneration gradual, and there is some sympathy in the recognition that many of Theodore's lies are ones he cannot help telling; but the final effect is devastatingly and unremittingly hostile. After Wells had replied to Louie to tell her of her mistake, scribbling on her letter 'this lady is a mythomaniac', she tried in an embarrassed second communication to explain herself by saying that she had been badly affected by the 'dreadful spate of notoriety' which had followed Lawrence's death, and by adding 'Your book seemed such a healthy cleanly analysis, after the hateful biographies that have been poured out'. She said that the novel had released feelings she did not know she possessed and then claimed, just as Jessie Chambers would have done, that 'being always torn with pity for [Lawrence], I never harboured bitterness'. Yet if it was not bitterness and resentment Louie harboured, and took with her to Vence, it would be hard to find alternative words for the feelings of anyone who could believe that Wells's 'healthy cleanly analysis' of the despicable Theodore Bulpington was also an analysis of Lawrence.

Nearer to the feelings of Ada than of Louie as they laid flowers on Lawrence's grave would have been those of Enid Hilton. She was the daughter of Willie Hopkin who had brought distinction to Eastwood by being able to entertain in his own home such figures of national importance as Keir Hardie, Ramsay MacDonald, and the Webbs. Although never much interested in socialism himself, Lawrence was fond of Hopkin and particularly of his wife Sallie, and spent many hours with them both discussing religion and politics. It was Hopkin who, on Lawrence's final visit to Eastwood in 1926, felt that he knew his young friend well enough to ask him why he had never married Jessie Chambers and who thereby elicited the response, 'It would have been a fatal step. I should have had too easy a life, nearly everything my own way, and my genius would have been destroyed.'

After she had married, Hopkin's daughter Enid was unusual for her time in spending all her holidays on trips abroad. When, as was often the case, the countries or towns she and her husband wanted to visit were ones Lawrence knew well, he would send her detailed instructions about the best routes to take and the most comfortable (and inexpensive) places to stay, demonstrating as he so often did that, had he not been a writer, he would have made a first-class travel agent. In return, and with something of her parents' spirited independence, Enid smuggled copies of *Lady Chatterley's Lover* into England, hiding them in her capacious knickers, so that they could then be sent to subscribers. The news of Lawrence's death she describes as a 'terrible shock'— 'I felt as half my life had passed away with him'—and she and her husband made their way to Vence as quickly as their respective jobs allowed. They found when they arrived that the Villa Robermond was already full of visitors but that Frieda had arranged for them to stay in a cottage nearby. The only visitor Enid Hilton identifies is Orioli but since he and Norman Douglas usually travelled together, this is likely to be the occasion when Douglas 'strewed a few red carnations on [Lawrence's] grave at Vence—an inoffensive gesture' (why he thought the qualification necessary is not clear). They had gone in a group to the cemetery and as they came away Enid remembered feeling very sad and trying not to cry. In order to lighten the mood, Orioli ushered them all into a café where, after some discussion with the waiter, he ordered a special liqueur to go with the coffee. The effect of this drink was, in Enid's words, to transform a number of 'misery-racked individuals into a happy laughing small crowd unable to control their mirth'. She had felt that Lawrence would not have liked her to cry but did not ask herself what he would have thought of her particular funeral party beginning to resemble an Irish wake. People laugh on solemn occasions because a long period of constrained gloom is unnatural for them; there may also be an element of hysteria in their laughter; and where death is involved laughter sometimes expresses a frank, animal satisfaction in still being alive when someone else is not. But it is true also that not everyone in Enid's party was as sad to lose Lawrence as she was. Most people liked Orioli and assumed that his relationship with Lawrence had been a warm and happy one. Yet when he came to write his memoirs he declared that on the whole it had been unsatisfactory, and complained that Lawrence could be very troublesome in business matters and was above all disconcertingly unpredictable. 'I wonder how many of those who knew him well were really sorry when he died,' he wrote, implicitly placing himself in the category of those who were not and almost certainly including in it also Norman Douglas, who was generally thought to have helped Orioli a good deal with the composition of his memoir.

We can be fairly certain that, in contrast to Orioli and Douglas, Enid Hilton was sorry when Lawrence died and she later showed her commitment by acting as Aldous Huxley's unpaid secretary when he was putting together the 1932 collection of Lawrence's letters. This was working to preserve the memory of the dead and a way of keeping it alive in herself although, as Proust points out, those memories of dead loved ones which matter most are likely to be involuntary. Because of what he calls the intermittences of the heart, and a failure of coincidence between the calendar of events and that of the feelings, Proust's narrator is relatively unmoved by the death of his grandmother, even though he has previously been devoted to her. It is only a year later, when he returns to the seaside town he had first visited with her, that he is suddenly overwhelmed by a sense of her loss and racked with guilt at the thought of remarks he had once made which upset her. He welcomes this experience as a salvation from hardness of heart or what he calls *la sécheresse de l'âme*. There were many moments after Lawrence's death when Frieda's return to places she had previously visited in his company must have brought back involuntary memories of him. If she did not cherish them with the same intensity as Proust's Marcel, it was because his eyes are firmly directed towards the past whereas she was someone with an unusual capacity, which her husband had always admired, for making the most of the here and now, and looking forward with optimism to the future.

Part III

Remembrance

16

Will-Power

Death renders us powerless but human beings have always sought ways of mitigating that unfortunate fact. One of the most important of these is the last will and testament. Making a will is a method for extending one's influence beyond the grave familiar to us from major fictional examples such as that in Shakespeare's *Merchant of Venice*. The father of Portia, with the anxiety concerning single women of independent means characteristic of the Elizabethans, has devised elaborate means for ensuring that she should bestow her hand (and fortune) appropriately. It seems right that, in the casket scenes, Portia should regularly be played as keener to obey the letter of her father's will than its spirit since the efforts of the dying to determine the future are often frustrated. Shakespeare himself made a will in which his financial assets, property, and household goods were not divided equally between his two daughters, and certainly not between those daughters and his wife, but were almost all given to his elder child Susanna with the proviso that they should then percolate down the centuries through the most nearly related male. The intention was to found 'a line' but biology cannot be predicted and by the end of the seventeenth century there were no direct descendants to whom his carefully preserved estate could pass.

Of all the wills of literary figures, Shakespeare's is the best known. Lawrence was in no position to compete since he did not leave a will at all but died, as the lawyers say, intestate. This is surprising given the sense of ultra responsibility he often displayed in financial matters. After he and Frieda had left New Mexico their ranch was occupied for a while by his fervent admirer, the Honourable Dorothy Brett. She had a modest private income but was careless about money and confessed in a letter that she had given to a local storekeeper a cheque which she knew would bounce. Lawrence was appalled. 'I would be loathe to draw a cheque if I thought it wouldn't be covered,' he lectured her, 'it's sort of false.' When he was penniless during the war he accumulated a number of small debts, the more personal of which he was afterwards very anxious to pay back; and when later he managed the sale of *Lady Chatterley's Lover* to subscribers, he was scrupulous about keeping accounts (too scrupulous in the opinion of Orioli, whose attitude may have partly been determined by his having agreed to take only 10 per cent of the profits while Lawrence took the other 90). It seems uncharacteristic of a man who, without ever being mean, was a meticulous manager of his own affairs that he should not have made arrangements for how they should be disposed of after his death. His nephew Ernest, the son of his surviving brother George, claimed that Lawrence held an old Arab belief that making a will is a recipe for imminent death; but Ernest was a notoriously unreliable witness who would later tell people that his uncle was such a keen supporter of Mussolini that he had been personally invited to come and live in Italy by the Italian dictator when he came to power in 1922. (Lawrence in fact disapproved of

Mussolini and after a demented Irishwoman's attempt at assassination only succeeded in leaving the Duce with a damaged nose, unsympathetically remarked that now he could put a ring through it.) A more likely explanation for the absence of a will than Ernest's is that Lawrence did not expect to die so soon, familiar as he was with narrow escapes.

Making no will would not have mattered in the early days when Lawrence had nothing to leave. After the dire poverty of the war his fortunes had improved in the early 1920s, yet by the time he was busy with the first two versions of *Lady Chatterley's Lover* he was complaining that he was still poor despite a lifetime of literary effort. It is possible that, in his anxiety to secure his own future but more particularly Frieda's, one of the motives Lawrence had for writing that novel as he finally did can be found in his realization that there were rich rewards for notoriety in the world in which he lived. *Lady Chatterley's Lover* was an undoubted financial success but his literary agent in England was worried that the attention it brought him might damage his career. The effect seems to have been the opposite and he found himself in his final years more in demand than ever before, among magazine editors but more significantly in the highly profitable world of newspaper journalism. The result was that, when he died, Frieda was able to report there was around £4,000 in investments or in the bank. This was not a fortune but in a period when the purchasing power of the pound was about forty times what it is now, neither was it small beer.

What Frieda quickly discovered was that this money was not all hers. As the widow of a man who had died intestate, she was entitled to £1,000, a life interest on the whole of her husband's estate and 'personal chattels', a phrase which mainly referred to those household accessories and furnishings which Lawrence in his peripatetic life had always made a point of not accumulating. All this was better than the second-best bed, but rather less than Frieda must have hoped for. In the period immediately following her husband's death, Ida Rauh lent her money and Huxley took care of the immediate funeral expenses, but then another and quite unexpected call on her resources came from the illness of her daughter Barbara. This was first diagnosed as tuberculosis of the spine and her neck was put in a cast. A little later she began to show signs of the severe mental derangement which led to her wild behaviour at the door of the room where Lawrence had died and she would abuse her mother with 'You fool, you fool'. As the condition developed into full-scale lunacy, Barby would throw off all her clothes, dabble in her own excrement, physically assault Frieda, or sit for hours making curious winding movements with her arms. The diagnosis of the doctor was now hysteria and his astonishing advice that what the young woman required was a man ('il lui faut un mâle'). Her mother found a local workman in whom Barby had shown some interest and who was willing to sleep with her, but the improvement was only temporary. When afterwards news of these events leaked out, it was assumed that Frieda had been following in a besotted manner what she imagined were Lawrentian principles whereas in fact she is more likely to have been the victim of an ancient prejudice in the medical profession that female hysteria is always a result of sexual frustration. In despair, she took Barby to another doctor whose verdict was that her daughter had syphilis of the brain. Given that after Frieda had been forced to send Barby back to her relations in England in the company of a nurse, she made a rapid and complete recovery and then lived into her eighties, neither tuberculosis of the bone nor syphilis seem likely explanations of what was wrong with her; but her behaviour in Vence not only caused her mother great distress but also considerable expense. In the account which she gave of the whole episode to Mabel Luhan in 1931, and which Mabel seems to have taken down almost verbatim before passing it on to her friend Una Jeffers, Frieda describes how the full-time nurse she had hired was sometimes obliged to hold Barby down on her bed. After one of these episodes the nurse said, 'When Mademoiselle has days like this I must be paid double.' 'Oh, what you cost me Barby, in that year!' was then Frieda's comment.

The difficulty about money emerges most clearly in Frieda's correspondence with the publisher of the Paris edition of *Lady Chatterley's Lover*, Edward Titus. The book was still doing well but Titus was reluctant to pay royalties until he was certain of the legal position. On the advice of Huxley, and very shortly after Lawrence's death, Frieda went to London and applied for the 'letters of administration' which would allow her to manage her late husband's ongoing literary affairs. Since the other party with an interest in the estate was the Lawrence family, the person appointed to administer it in conjunction with Frieda was his brother George. This was almost certainly a consequence of his being the oldest of Lawrence's surviving siblings rather than a question of gender, but it was nevertheless a strange choice. A wild youth who had to be bought out of the army by his mother when he was 19 and whose girlfriend was three months pregnant when he married her, George developed into an eminently respectable citizen, a lay preacher and teetotaller who had strongly disapproved of his brother's relationship with Frieda. Becoming a co-administrator brought him into contact or, in some cases, allowed him to renew contact with many of Lawrence's English friends, including Lady Ottoline Morrell. 'Over six foot, tall stately woman, one of the Bentincks you know', is how he described her during a recorded interview made late in his life and he went on to recount that, when they were once in a car together, she put her hand on his knee and asked, 'George, do you agree with Frieda's attitude to sex?' 'I most certainly do not,' he replied, to which Lady Ottoline then responded, 'Good man, neither do I.' One has to hear George Lawrence's Nottinghamshire accent, and imagine Lady Ottoline's upper-class one, to have the full flavour of this anecdote. It was not until October 1930 that Titus received from George a letter authorizing him to deal with Frieda directly in the matter of the royalties and having to consult in all her other literary dealings someone so fundamentally unsympathetic to what she felt Lawrence represented was a legal obligation she came more and more to resent.

That there were a lot of these dealings was a result of Lawrence having died at the height of his fame or notoriety. After the publication of *Lady Chatterley's Lover* had come the closure of his London exhibition of paintings by the police and, in between these two events, questions had been asked in Parliament about a registered package containing a typescript of *Pansies* which the authorities had seized as it arrived in Britain from the South of France. Everyone knew who Lawrence was and immediately following his death publishers and literary agents gathered around Frieda like bees round a honey-pot. Titus was one of those who made the loudest buzz, begging her for any unpublished material and claiming to have found someone in London willing to offer her £500 for the right to publish *Apocalypse*, his short work on the Book of Revelation. This was a very large sum for a book of minority interest and Frieda must have regretted being unable to profit from it; but she had already given *Apocalypse* to Orioli along with *The Virgin and the Gipsy*, that splendid example of the novella form which Lawrence practised as successfully as any other writer in English. The virgin of its title was clearly based on Barbara Weekley and it was she who provided many intimate details of the relations her father had sent her to live with after Frieda had left him. Lawrence used these to evoke a potent atmosphere of domestic staleness and restriction in the middle of which he placed a satirical portrait of Frieda's former husband as the Reverend Saywell, mealy-mouthed, conventional, and fundamentally ignorant of his own nature. The virgin's escape from this environment is effected by not only the gipsy she meets but also a cleansing flood, and in his description of both, Lawrence manoeuvres so skilfully between realism and allegory that when at the beginning of 1926 he had completed the work, he must have been pleased with the results. Uncharacteristically, he then declined to publish, saying only of the Reverend Saywell that he was after all Barby's father. Lawrence clearly felt some compunction about exposing the Weekley family to scorn and he may also have feared there could be legal complications. When afterwards he occasionally talked of 'revising' *The Virgin and the Gipsy* it would not be because he felt it was carelessly written (the reverse is the case), but that he needed to make its sources in real life less obvious. Frieda felt no such need, and no anxiety about the consequences for her former husband or for Barby of the story's appearance; but after she had arranged for the publication of both *Apocalypse* and *The Virgin and the Gipsy* with Orioli (probably during the visit to Vence which Enid Hilton remembered) she must have realized that she was acting illegally. To Titus therefore she said that Lawrence had given *Apocalypse* to her before he died, with the injunction to do what she liked with it; and that it was also before his death that he had already made arrangements with Orioli for the publication of *The Virgin*. There is no evidence for the truth of either claim.

Past and future publications of her husband's work, with their associated royalties, were not Frieda's only concern. Lawrence may not have left many 'personal chattels' of the conventional kind but there were a good number of paintings and even more manuscripts. The paintings she had sent to Vence and with the help of a friend called Martha Crotch, who ran a pottery and antique shop within the walls of the town, held an exhibition in the hope of attracting buyers. Potential buyers of the manuscripts were more easily forthcoming. Lawrence had only begun to be properly conscious of the value of his manuscripts in the early 1920s. When in 1924 Mabel Luhan had wanted to give him the small ranch above Taos which she owned, she decided to give it instead to Frieda because she knew how fiercely he disliked being under an obligation. Not to be manipulated in this way, Lawrence made a present to Mabel of a manuscript of *Sons and Lovers*. This may have struck her as a token gesture at the time but since the ranch was small and dilapidated, there could have been something in Frieda's later contention that Mabel received more than she gave in the exchange. In 1928 Harry Crosby offered five gold $20 pieces for a manuscript of the short story 'Sun'. This had been lost but Lawrence ensured there was a sale by writing out the story again, making it in the process more erotic, and then always referring to this version subsequently as 'unexpurgated'. The following year, when Dorothy Brett was living on the ranch, it was falsely reported to the Lawrences that she was meeting her extra expenses by selling off manuscripts which had been left there. Writing to explain how angry he would feel if this were true, Lawrence told Brett that he kept the manuscripts as a 'sort of nest-egg', that he depended on them for 'his reserve'. In 1930 they became Frieda's reserve and while she was in London securing the letters of administration she had discussions with at least one possible buyer. At that time she said she would sell all of them for £25,000. This was regarded as a wildly unrealistic figure but it would be interesting to know what the legal position would have been of any sum she had then managed to negotiate. In the wording of the legislation which governed her position (the Administration of Estates Act of 1925), paintings were included among 'personal chattels' but there was no mention of a dead author's manuscripts and all those chattels were excluded which were being 'used at the death of the intestate for business purposes'.

In the difficulties which Frieda soon began to experience with her co-administrator George, Ada resolutely took her side. It would be an understatement to say that the two women had not always got on. When at the beginning of 1926 the Lawrences were in Spotorno on the Italian Riviera, renting the villa which belonged to Angelo Ravagli's wife, Ada visited them. Because her brother was ill, she seems to have taken over the responsibility of nursing and so comprehensively that on one occasion Frieda found the bedroom door locked against her. There was a great deal of friction between all three parties and it was partly to avoid it that, when he was feeling better, Lawrence went to Capri where he met up with Dorothy Brett and made a failed attempt at a sexual relationship which was highly distressing to them both. Frieda meanwhile stayed in Spotorno and began or perhaps merely continued her affair with Ravagli. By this time Ada was back in her home at Ripley, just over the Nottinghamshire border into Derbyshire; but she was too fond of her brother to bear any grudges once he had become reconciled with Frieda and a visit she made to Bandol at the beginning of 1929 seems to have gone well. After Lawrence had died she set herself against her sister Emily, her brother George, and all the other members of the Lawrence family in firmly insisting that Frieda should have everything. Better off than either of her siblings but also a woman of fierce integrity, Ada was only concerned to do what she believed her brother would have wanted; and she must largely have based her conduct on a letter he had sent to her in September 1929. This dealt with what Lawrence called the 'final disposal' of his books and pictures, about which he insisted he was not all sentimental. He was hanging on to them at present, he went on, because they represented his capital but in any case he had 'no use for family and heirlooms'. To explain why this should be so he simply reminded Ada that 'George is the head of the "family", if you talk of family' and that George's son Ernest was therefore 'the legal heir of heirlooms'. If he died, he wrote, in a very rare use of that phrase, 'the mss and pictures would have to be sold to secure something of an income for Frieda'. Written less than six months before he had in fact died the letter was clearly crucial for Ada and she willingly participated in the scheme Frieda had developed by September 1930 to persuade Lawrence's brother and sisters to sign a paper saying that all they wanted from the estate was a reversion of copyright to the family after her death. But Emily and George failed to cooperate and a year later Frieda was calling George a calamity and complaining that he refused to pass royalties on to her because his only concern was 'to swell the estate'. There was clearly a conflict of interest between the two with Frieda wanting to realize as much capital as possible and George hoping perhaps to safeguard it for a time when she would no longer be there. A will would have resolved their difficulties but Frieda claimed that, although in his last hours or days Lawrence began to talk about the need to make one, she was so anxious to save him distress, and not to deprive him of hope, that she told him there was no need to bother. She would willingly have risked being a charwoman for the rest of her days, she boldly wrote to Emily later, than have done anything which would have given Lawrence five more minutes of trouble and misery.

17

Lying for Truth

Almost as soon as Frieda became aware of her likely legal difficulties, she was offered a potential escape from them by John Middleton Murry. Before their definitive break in the mid-1920s, Murry had been Lawrence's closest friend, his enthusiastic and sometimes slavish disciple. Leaving behind him a second wife who was soon to follow Katherine Mansfield in dying from tuberculosis, he came to Vence only a few weeks after Lawrence's death, to visit the grave perhaps, but also to see what he could do to help Frieda. It was after he had read to her from Lawrence's work in his beautiful voice, she later complained to Mabel Luhan, that he then made love to her but Mabel privately reflected that Frieda was rather too old a hand to decline any responsibility for being 'seduced'. Murry himself said that with Frieda, and for the first time in his life, he knew what fulfilment in love really meant.

This episode was the culmination of a process which had begun as far back as the winter of 1923. Lawrence was then in Mexico, temporarily separated from Frieda, who had insisted on returning to Europe to see her children. Wanting also to see her mother, she had travelled to Germany in the company of Murry, who (in his account) had regretfully refused her offer of a sexual relationship out of loyalty to her husband. Once Lawrence had rejoined Frieda in Europe, he wrote several stories in which Murry very obviously figured and in which he revealed his suspicion (or perhaps knowledge) that there had been more intimacy between his wife and supposed best friend than he liked. The strangest and most remarkable of these is called 'The Border-Line'. The heroine of this story, who is unmistakably Frieda, has been married to a soldier who has been declared missing during the war and is equally unmistakably Lawrence. She is now married to a man who was her first husband's friend and happens to have all the physical characteristics of Murry. As the heroine starts to feel the difference between her previous union with a 'born fighter, a sword not to be sheathed', and marriage to 'this other man, this cunning civilian, this subtle equivocator, this adjuster of the scales of truth', she also begins to catch glimpses of her dead husband's ghost. In the climax of the story, her resurrected first husband infects his successor with tuberculosis and pushes him out of the heroine's bed just as she is about to offer him some physical comfort. He then makes love to her himself but in a manner which, while it seems to exclude penetration, crushes her 'in the last, final ecstasy of submission'. Murry's sexual relations with Frieda in 1930 were no doubt more conventional and there is no record of any ghost of her late husband coming back from the dead to prevent them.

The escape Murry offered Frieda when he came to Vence lay in a reminder that Lawrence had once made a will in which he left everything to her. In the winter of 1914, Murry encouraged Frieda to recall, he and Katherine Mansfield had been living close to the Lawrences at Chesham in Buckinghamshire. With the war just begun, the two men decided to make wills in which they left everything to their partners and then to have the resulting documents witnessed by each other. Before Murry's 1930 visit, Frieda makes no mention of there ever having been a will and it was only after it that she began to claim that there had been one which was lost during the removal from New Mexico. Whenever she later wrote about how this will was drawn up, she placed the episode in Cornwall in 1916 rather than in Buckinghamshire almost two years earlier. But memory is fallible. The idea of even a lost will was important because it offered proof of Lawrence's intentions and opened what was at least the possibility of pushing George out of the picture.

Frieda became increasingly keen to do exclude George because she increasingly felt the need for money. Barby's illness was one reason for this but another and more important one was the plan she had to retreat to the ranch in New Mexico with Angelo Ravagli. When the Lawrences were staying in Spotorno, their stove began to smoke and in his capacity as their landlady's husband Ravagli came round to fix it. He did this so effectively that Lawrence observed that he would be a good man to have with one back at the ranch. Frieda always took this casual remark as an endorsement of her scheme to take Angelo with her to New Mexico but there were considerable difficulties in her path. The most obvious of these was Signora Ravagli and her three children. Frieda was godmother to the youngest child and tried to keep up relations with all the Ravagli family. In the early summer of 1931 she invited mother and children to stay with her in her rented house in Vence—no longer the Villa Robermond because that had been felt to be too full of memories of Lawrence painful to Barby. After entertaining them for a while, Frieda left for New Mexico while Ravagli, who was not then in Vence, took six months unpaid leave from his regiment in order to join her. Her friend Martha Crotch was left to manage the situation. She felt that Ravagli's wife understood how invidious her position had become when she let 'two fat tears' drop as she was explaining that her husband had gone to the States 'to help Madame Lawrence on the *ferme*'.

Angelo was Frieda's lover but he also provided an indispensable help to her on the ranch. She could not have managed without him. On their first arrival she bought a car which he could drive and it seemed obvious that she would have to compensate him for his lack of income from the army. As he busily began to make living conditions on the ranch more comfortable, there were a lot of additional expenses. These seemed to have coincided with the increasing difficulties with George and strengthened Frieda's resolve to secure untrammelled access to the whole of her husband's estate principally by playing the card of the lost will. Her new life with Angelo needed financing, especially if it was to continue, as she very much hoped, beyond the initial six months.

In societies where women rarely go out to work, widowhood can bring with it a dramatic loss of status. Those who had seemed to be friends of the couple turn out to have been friends of the husband only; the widow is gradually dropped from the social circles to which she and her husband once belonged; and there is a tendency to forget that she still exists. Frieda was not of the stamp to suffer this kind of fate. When in her relations with Lady Ottoline Morrell during the war, she felt she had detected an inclination not to treat her as her husband's equal but rather as some inconvenient appendage, she had reacted violently. But there was no need for violent reaction when she returned to London in 1932 to pursue her legal claims because the majority of Lawrence's former friends made her welcome and she was lionized as the widow of a famous writer. It was not only literary agents and potential publishers who wined and dined her but eminent figures from the literary world such as George Bernard Shaw. Frieda basked in the attention she received and helped to ensure its continuance, not only by the strength of her personality but also by always suggesting that Lawrence's works were almost as much hers as his. What she meant by this was that meeting her had saved Lawrence from being a psychological wreck and allowed him to pursue his literary career; that they always discussed his writings together; and that many of them were in any case based on her experience both before and after her marriage to him. (In an extraordinary extension of this last claim she had on her return to the ranch told Mabel Luhan that parts of *Lady Chatterley's Lover* had been inspired by Lawrence's knowledge of her affair with Angelo.) Without her, the story ran, there would have been no great writer and, as her legal troubles with George increased, she made a particular point of contemptuously dismissing any notion that a contribution could have been made to that greatness by Lawrence's family. This greatly distressed Ada, as did the abuse of George and Emily contained in the letters she now began to receive from Frieda. Lawrence and Frieda were neither of them temperate people, as their famous quarrels illustrated; but her tendency for jumping to conclusions and flying off the handle was even greater than his. In her dealings with members of her husband's family, she also displayed an especially wounding talent for remembering the uncomplimentary remarks which their brother had occasionally launched in their direction, and not failing to report them.

In the summer of 1932 Ada was refusing to communicate further with Frieda but still determined to support her right to the whole of her brother's estate. She made one last effort to avoid legal proceedings by reintroducing the idea that George and Emily should sign a document stating that all they wanted was a reversion of the copyrights to them after Frieda's death, and she reinforced her position as a disinterested broker by insisting that for herself or her own family she wanted nothing. But a solution which would have been welcomed by Frieda in 1930 was now no longer acceptable. What her lawyers did was offer Lawrence's brother and elder sister each a sum of money, and one or two pictures and manuscripts, in exchange for which they were to drop any claim whatsoever. She told Ada that it was her siblings who had themselves asked for £700 each but this, Ada insisted, was a deliberate lie. According to her, the initiative had come from Frieda's side and her literary agent Pollinger had travelled up to Nottingham with signed cheques for £500 in his pocket and dire warnings about the legal costs if Emily and George chose to fight the case through the courts. Outraged, Ada declared that accepting what was after all their brother's money so that Frieda could be 'rid of the family' would be a disgrace for them all and later noted that the solution she had been proposing was one supported by Huxley, Orioli, and all Lawrence's 'real friends'. But her pleas fell on deaf ears.

That Emily and George agreed to settle took away any adversarial element in the hearing which was eventually held in early November 1932 and which became a rubber-stamping of what had already been agreed. The court accepted the contention of Mr Bucknill, Frieda's barrister, that there had once been a 1914 will similar to the one, signed by Lawrence and Frieda, which Murry had made on 9 November of that year in favour of Katherine Mansfield. Bucknill's willingness to ascribe a precise date to this document strongly suggests he must have seen it, but no one else mentions having done so and of course its existence in no way proved that there had ever been an equivalent will made by Lawrence. The case for being sceptical about the story Frieda and Murry told does not only rely on her failure to mention a will before his Vence visit and her continuing confusion about details thereafter, nor on the suggestion that if Frieda's solicitor had been confident of his case, he might not have felt the need to buy off George and Emily. There is also the absence in the surviving documentation relating to November 1914 of any reference to a supposed will-making, even though both Murry and Mansfield kept private diaries throughout that month. But perhaps the most crucial items of evidence are phrases from a letter which Lawrence wrote to his friend Catherine Carswell in October 1921. He was not then very busy, he told her, 'just pottering with short stories', and he went on: 'Think I may as well get the mss together as far as possible. Feel like making my will also. Not that I'm going to die. But to give myself a nice sense of finality.' The three possible explanations of: 'Feel like making my will also' seem to be that Lawrence had forgotten he had already made one; that he did not take the one he had made in 1914 seriously; or, much more probably, that he had never made a will at all.

There may of course have been some talk of will-making between the Lawrences, Murry, and Katherine Mansfield in

1914 even though Mansfield was the only one of the quartet who at that period had anything to leave (in the will she made before she died in 1923, she left Lawrence a book about which he was never told and which he certainly never received). It is possible also that there was some foundation to the story Frieda told the court of a document which she had glimpsed when she was packing to leave the ranch in 1925 and which was subsequently lost. But if the story of the 1914 will was indeed partly or largely a concoction, it would have been regarded by Murry, and more especially by Frieda, as a case of lying for truth. As the woman who had lived with Lawrence for close on twenty years, she always felt she knew what he had really intended. The trouble was that Ada acted from an identical conviction, sure in her own mind that she knew what her brother would have wanted. In the absence of documentation, there was no one able to arbitrate their dispute except the husband and brother who had now crossed the borderline for good.

Frieda felt exultant after the settlement. She had been anxious that she would be harshly treated and was gratified by the respect the judge showed to her and to the memory of her husband. Her anxiety was perhaps a little unnecessary in that the gamble of a court case had been replaced by what was perhaps the greater gamble of giving money to George and Emily. One thousand pounds was a large sum to find, there were her own high legal costs, and part of the deal may have involved her meeting theirs. But Frieda calculated that the demand for Lawrence's work would continue and she was proved right. With money from the estate she was able to provide Angelo with a monthly income so that he could leave the army and live with her permanently in New Mexico. Together they renovated the ranch, building a new house on the same site and farming on a very modest scale although eventually Frieda bought another, additional ranch house further down the mountain where conditions were less primitive and harsh. They spent many of their first winters in California, where the Huxleys had gone to live, but after Frieda had acquired a third property near Brownsville on the Gulf of Mexico, they often went there. Royalties from Lawrence's books and the occasional sale of a manuscript did not make them rich but it left them comfortably off, even during the years of the Depression. The one disappointment from a financial point of view was the collection of Lawrence's paintings. Frieda had probably asked too much for these and, after the interest shown by the Aga Khan, they found no buyers. In 1936 she was obliged to ship them over from Vence to a special room Angelo had prepared in what became known as the 'upper ranch'. Apart from an early and brief appearance of one or two to them in an exhibition in Los Angeles (where none was sold), they stayed in this room until Frieda's death in 1956 after which they fell into the hands of a local Greek hotelier who at one point declared that he would be willing to return them to England if the British government would send the Elgin marbles back to Greece. There were limited opportunities in Taos for exhibiting them and they seem to have attracted little interest although it may be that, with enough money to live on, Frieda was not very interested in a sale. She was not fundamentally a mercenary woman. No one who had left a university professor of foreign languages for a virtually penniless working-class writer whose health was poor could have been that.

Dr Johnson writes interestingly about a friend of his who had an incurably sick wife and had to do all the nursing himself because he was so short of money. He conjectures that this friend 'probably thought often how lightly he should tread the path of life without his burden' and adds, 'Of this thought the admission was unavoidable, and the indulgence might be forgiven to frailty and distress'. Life for Frieda in the final months or even years of Lawrence's life had not been easy and there must have been some relief when his sufferings were finally over. Her temperament meant that, once he was gone, she could tread the path of life lightly and with only minimum compunction. On her first return to the ranch with Angelo in 1931, she held a party where couples danced to gramophone records, there were lanterns in the trees, and a banner between them read 'Una noce in Venezia'. Whereas Queen Victoria preserved her consort's clothes and famously had them laid out every morning long after his death, it did not trouble Frieda that Angelo should make use of a pair of her dead husband's trousers which had been left at the ranch, even if—bought for a much thinner man—they did not button at the waist. (It was when she caught sight of Angelo in Lawrence's trousers that Dorothy Brett was strengthened in her conviction that she was Lorenzo's real widow.) Frieda had turned 50 in 1929 but friends who saw her on her return to London in 1932 were struck by how happy she looked, and also how youthful. At her husband's funeral she had scandalized a few of the more conventional inhabitants of Vence by wearing a silk dress of scarlet and gold. When she had first bought it, Lawrence had told her that it would suit her better if she were a year or two younger. That is how she now appeared to many friends, several among whom would have associated her rejuvenated appearance with having a lover twelve years her junior. To have replaced

Lawrence so quickly, and to be living her new life on the proceeds of his labours, were matters which she handled with such statements as 'When you have been married to a Lawrence, you can't be put on the shelf'. She wanted the approval of her dead husband and was fortunate in always believing that she would have had it. Occasional moments of doubt she was able to brush aside. In the late 1930s, for example, Frieda negotiated the sale of a manuscript of *Sons and Lovers* which had annotations in the hand of Jessie Chambers. She hoped it would go to a nice person because of 'the Miriam bits in it' (Miriam being the name in the novel of the Jessie Chambers figure), and said that she would like to burn all the manuscripts because she knew how Lawrence had hated 'the personal touch'. She then added, in the inconsequential manner characteristic of her, 'But I daresay he wanted me to have the money'. Shortly before she died in 1956, she remarked to her sister Else that it had been 'a very good year financially' and that she had never thought she would have been on 'such a green branch'. 'I know', she went on, 'Lorenzo would not begrudge it me.' The branch in question was of course about to become spectacularly greener with the *Lady Chatterley* trial. By the terms of Frieda's will half the royalties which that event generated went to her three children by Weekley while the other half went to Angelo and the wife and children he had by then rejoined in Italy. The bargain struck in 1932 meant that members of the Lawrence family continued to receive nothing at all.

18

Image Rights

In one of the more accessible sections of *Being and Nothingness*, Jean-Paul Sartre sets out to refute what he believed was Heidegger's approach to death. His objection is to a way of thinking that encourages people to compare dying to the last note in a melody, one which retrospectively confers meaning and coherence on all that has gone before. Sartre wants instead to reaffirm the arbitrary and (as he puts it) *absurd* nature of death. It is not only 'the project which destroys all projects . . . the impossible destruction of my expectations', but also 'the triumph of the point of view of the Other' over any image people might harbour of themselves. He does not deny that there is life after death but it is a life 'of which the Other makes himself the guardian'. A little later he writes, less comfortingly, 'To be dead is to be the prey for the living.'

A person's image represents their meaning in the world but it might reasonably be objected here that we all of us have a great deal of difficulty in establishing that meaning when we are alive, never mind when we are dead; and that too often we are reduced to the querulous complaint of the woman in T. S. Eliot's *Prufrock*: 'That is not it at all | That is not what I meant, at all.' Sartre retorts by pointing out that at least when we are living we are in a position to battle against other people's views of ourselves whereas death

gives 'the final victory to the point of view of the Other by ...
suddenly suppressing one of the combatants'. We do certainly live
on in the minds of others and are thus able to 'pursue (our) history
in the human world', but it is only as what Sartre calls 'objective
and opaque beings'. Death deprives us 'of all subjective meaning
in order to hand (us) over to any objective meaning which the
Other is pleased to give'. A simplified paraphrase of his position
might be that death takes away our power and delivers us
powerless into the hands of what it is convenient to call posterity.

Making a will can be construed as one method for trying to
escape this powerlessness but so too can the provision which
important people from the past sometimes made to have a
monument erected to their memory, one by which their image, in
the primary sense of that word, could be perpetuated. The second
Earl of Southampton for example, father of the Southampton to
whom Shakespeare dedicated *Venus and Adonis* and *The Rape of
Lucrece*, left elaborate instructions for the completion of his
monument together with legacies to his dependents which would
have demonstrated the generosity of his nature. But he
compromised the quality of his posthumous fame by also leaving
too little money to cover the proposed expenses. Caring about how
people will think of us once we are dead seems a confirmation of
Freud's contention that it is impossible for most people to imagine
their own non-existence, and that whatever post-mortem scenarios
they conjure up will always include themselves as hidden
spectators. Writers appear no more immune from making this
mistake than everyone else and many of them have thought
forward to a time when they and their work would be discussed,
as if what was then said could have some significance for their

decaying corpse. Burns, for example, was distressed as he was dying by not having been able to put his papers in order and by the knowledge that they contained many malicious squibs which were likely to be published after his death to the detriment of his reputation. There was no more determined materialist than Stendhal but he worried about the after-life of his writings and made a series of *testaments* which are only half-humorous and through which he hoped to ensure that his unpublished manuscripts fell into the right hands. What was said about their author might not have concerned him unduly, but in Stevenson's one and only will elaborate arrangements were made for ensuring that the right person would write his life and, absenting himself from felicity awhile, be the Horatio to his Hamlet. Suspicious of even 'authorized' biography, some writers have made sure they wrote their own life stories before they died. The champion in this area is Thomas Hardy who wrote an account of his life in the third person and then arranged that, after his death, it should be published by his widow under her name. He wanted to be certain that people should see him as he chose to be seen. But authorized biography of whatever kind always raises suspicion and does not in any case preclude rival biographies, once the documents are available or even when strenuous efforts have been made to conceal or destroy them.

Lawrence made no attempt to combat the widely held view that he was an unusually autobiographical novelist. When asked for details of his early life, he would cheerfully refer the enquirer to the first part of *Sons and Lovers*. Yet in his last years he wrote a number of non-fictional autobiographical sketches in which the image he presents of himself is different from that in the novel. Paul Morel is fundamentally his mother's boy. He identifies with her middle-class aspirations and joins her in despising the coarseness of her collier husband. But after *Sons and Lovers* was published, and even before, Lawrence came to feel that his excessive attachment to his mother had been damaging and began switching his adherence from her values to those of his father. In the late autobiographical sketches he writes of himself as an ordinary working-class boy with an instinctive sympathy for his father's world. It is this which has prevented him from 'getting on' as his mother so desperately desired he should, and which has meant that he is now isolated and *déclassé*, alienated from the bourgeoisie but too highly educated to live comfortably among the industrial working classes.

Lawrence seems to have elaborated this new image of himself chiefly for his own benefit. Members of the public would have begun to be aware of it from reading the introduction he wrote for his *Collected Poems* in 1928, some of his *Pansies*, the 'Autobiographical Sketch' in the volume of *Assorted Articles* published shortly after his death, or the essay 'Nottingham and the Mining Countryside' which appeared in the June 1930 number of the *New Adelphi* dedicated to his memory. But several of the more explicitly autobiographical pieces remained unpublished. He would have had no motive for trying to ensure he was correctly viewed after his death because he had no immediate intention of dying. When he did in fact die, his later autobiographical writings or remarks provided useful items of information for the obituary writers but that did not mean that they accepted the way those items were interpreted. The dead are accorded many privileges but being able to impose their own view of themselves on the world they leave behind is not one of them. Whatever his reasons,

Lawrence was wise not to make the efforts Hardy did to convey a true picture of himself to posterity when its more probing participants will always bite the hand that feeds: take what they otherwise would not have known from the autobiographical record but then use it in ways of which the dead person would never have approved.

On the day following Lawrence's death an old friend of his called Douglas Goldring was in a Nice bar frequented by the Riviera correspondents of English and American newspapers. One of the correspondents was reading out passages from a much-thumbed copy of *Lady Chatterley's Lover* (freely available in France but not in England), and denouncing them as 'sheer muck'. Goldring told him that if he and his colleagues 'sent obituary messages describing Lawrence as a pornographer they would disgrace their profession and the papers which employed them'. The initial notices were in fact anodyne enough. Whether through malice or misunderstanding, a false report circulated that the news of Lawrence's death had been kept secret by his friends, as if they had something shameful to hide; but otherwise the details of his life and career were in the first instance reported in a relatively neutral manner. He was a figure who attracted worldwide interest and responses to his death were therefore varied; but a majority of the notices shared several common features. One was an emphasis on his working-class background; another a reference, more or less extended or informed, to his lifelong struggle with poor health; and a third an account of his battle with the censors, from the time *The Rainbow* was banned during the war but with a stress more particularly on the recent trouble over *Lady Chatterley's Lover* and the paintings. A fourth common feature was the admission that for all his shortcomings Lawrence was after all a genius. This was a word he had learnt to distrust. In the 'Autobiographical Sketch' which was included in *Assorted Articles,* and which had previously appeared in the *Sunday Dispatch* as 'Myself Revealed', he describes how he had given the manuscript of *The White Peacock* to Ford Madox Ford, who had told him it had every fault the English novel can have but that he nonetheless had GENIUS. 'This made me want to laugh,' Lawrence comments, 'it sounded so comical. In the early days they were always telling me I had got genius, as if to console me for not having their own incomparable advantages.' The shrewdness of this remark became evident as short notices of Lawrence's death were succeeded by longer, evaluative obituaries. A common pattern emerged in them which is best described by the title of the biography of Lawrence which Richard Aldington was to publish in 1950, *Portrait of a Genius, But* ... It immediately became possible to distinguish between the obituaries by observing how much emphasis their authors chose to place on the 'but'.

The London Establishment view was as usual represented by *The Times*, whose obituary appeared on 4 March. Its author agreed that Lawrence undoubtedly had genius and could create characters which were 'even obtrusively real'. There were passages of description in his work so fine that they commanded 'the admiration of people much of his work disgusts'. Yet as time went on, 'and his disease took firmer hold', he began to confuse 'decency with hypocrisy, and honesty with the free and public use of vulgar words' until 'not content with words, he turned to painting in order to exhibit more clearly still his contempt for all reticence'. The writer concluded that the struggle with the censors which had inevitably resulted from this attitude meant that

Lawrence missed his place 'among the very best which his genius might have won'.

The tone in *The Times* was very different from that adopted on the same day in the *Manchester Guardian*, a great *provincial* newspaper and one less conservative in every way. Appropriately enough, its obituarist laid much heavier emphasis on Lawrence's origins, claiming that he was 'early exposed to the life-killing conditions in which a mechanistic industrialism has entangled mankind'. This is what explains not only the attacks in his work on 'the blind mechanism of industry' but also his search among primitive communities for a 'unity of instinctive life, untainted by self-conscious thought'. It was in that search that he was able to exercise the 'extraordinary powers of sensuous divination' apparent in his descriptions of the natural world. So far so good, yet in describing the effect of industrialization on Lawrence the *Guardian* writer calls him 'a genius pain-obsessed beyond the possibility of humour or tolerance' and claims that, if he turned to nature, it was because his self-conscious mind found transient appeasement there from 'its hysteria and tortured bitterness'. That he was moreover so 'obsessed by the physical and so hostile to the conscious mind' meant that he could not create 'varied and subtle characters'. And yet he was a 'superbly equipped craftsman' and 'no writer since Tolstoy had wrestled more fiercely or significantly than Lawrence with the death in life from which he could not break free'. A comparison with Tolstoy is the highest praise a novelist can ever receive and the intentions of the writer in the *Manchester Guardian* were clearly friendlier than those of the writer in *The Times*; but with friends of that kind, Lawrence might have remarked, he would never need many enemies.

Enemies he nonetheless had in plenty. One of these was J. C. Squire, a prominent London writer and journalist whom Lawrence had publicly mocked in one of his poems and who published a long obituary in the *Observer* on 9 March. This began with the confident but quite false suggestion that before receiving what little ' "higher education" ' he could lay claim to, Lawrence had followed his father down the pit. Later works like *Lady Chatterley's Lover* Squire dismissed as unworthy of Lawrence's genius and the unavoidable consequence of 'some kind of galloping disease, whether consumption or another' (like the supposed secrecy of his death, 'or another' hints at the syphilis which in the conventional thinking of the time awaited all those over-concerned with sex). It might be felt, Squire implied, that allowances ought to be made for Lawrence's poor health and hopelessly disadvantaged social background, but 'even germs can work only upon the material they find already in existence'. Whereas the effect of consumption on Keats and Stevenson was to make them even more generous and affectionate, the consequences for someone as initially vain, self-centred, grudging, and morose as Lawrence were necessarily different. As for any social difficulties he may have encountered, many men had overcome worse without losing their faith, hope, and charity. Squire then went on for two pages complaining about Lawrence: that he was self-righteous and pontifical, for example, or without 'commonsense, humour, tenderness or understanding of human character'. It comes as a surprise therefore to find him concluding that 'at the climax of his powers, Lawrence, both in prose and verse, achieved things that no other writer has achieved' and finally suggesting that in his travel books and his poetry there are passages 'as vivid and illuminating as any that ever were written'. A genius then, yet one who is accompanied in Squire's mind by an exceptionally long and damaging list of qualifications.

The obituaries in *The Times,* the *Manchester Guardian* and the *Observer* were the opening salvoes in a particularly lively battle for image rights: for the privilege of informing the public what D. H. Lawrence was really like. He had not made that task easy by being someone who excited strong feelings of either liking or loathing but to whom it was hard to remain indifferent. The tone which prevailed in discussions of his death made his supporters angry. A pamphlet was published in response to the Squire obituary and Rhys Davies, the Welsh writer who had been with Lawrence on the trip from Bandol to Paris, spoke for many of the younger admirers when he said that the newspapers were full of 'such repetitions of revilings that one had the impression of a pack of evilly surly convicts released at last'. Because the tendency of even the more favourable notices was to represent Lawrence as a gloomy, obsessed neurotic, Murry wrote a letter to the *Times Literary Supplement* on 13 March in which he protested that his friend had not been 'a madman of genius' but rather 'the most remarkable and most lovable man [he] had ever known', and someone who was often gay. 'My dominant memory of him', he wrote, 'is of a blithe and joyful man.' The next day a letter from Catherine Carswell in *Time and Tide* insisted that Lawrence was not a 'morose, frustrated, tortured' person but 'gay, skilful, clever at everything'. Writing to the *Nation and Athenaeum* at the end of the month, E. M. Forster protested that now Lawrence was dead 'the low-brows whom he scandalized have united with the high-brows whom he bored to ignore his greatness' and he declared him 'the greatest imaginative novelist of his generation'. T. S. Eliot did not contest this judgement directly but he took the trouble of writing to the same journal a week later in order to suggest that Forster's claim was without meaning unless he could make clear to his reader exactly what he meant by 'greatest', 'imaginative', and 'novelist'. It was a pedantic challenge which Forster wisely chose to ignore.

To enforce his notion of the powerlessness of the dead, and the arbitrary and absurd nature of dying, Sartre offers the example of the young man who 'has lived for 30 years in the expectation of becoming a great writer'. When this young man then dies, having published only one book, 'suddenly the very expectation which he was, the expectation of being a great man, loses any kind of meaning'. While he was living, that expectation was either 'a vain and senseless obstinacy or a profound apprehension of his value'; but once he is deprived of the ability to write books, the final value and meaning of his conduct 'remains forever in suspense'. The point is obvious enough but it provides a useful reminder of the significance of quite when a writer dies. Because Keats died so young, commentators have found it impossible to refrain from speculating about what he might have become; and we are sometimes asked to imagine how differently we would regard George Eliot had she not survived middle age. That Lawrence died while the *Lady Chatterley* controversy was still raging was good for business but not perhaps for his future reputation. It meant that from the beginning there was a heavy stress on an aspect of his writing and career where he is not at his most impressive. Yet he had no more choice in the matter than the Lady Macbeth whose husband would have famously preferred her to have died 'hereafter'. Death comes how and when it will and immediately gives a final shape or pattern to a life which it never had before. In Lawrence's case it came after forty-four years. This makes him luckier than Jonathan Miller's 5-year-old son believed that he was when he was found by his father in a flood of tears and complaining, 'I don't want to die, I've not had a long enough turn yet'; but also less fortunate than H. G. Wells who, at a dinner given in honour of his seventieth birthday by the PEN club, said that he felt like 'a little boy at a lovely party, who has been given quite a lot of lovely toys and who has spread his play about the floor. Then comes his nurse. "Now Master Bertie", she says, "it's getting late. Time you began to put away your toys."' Several of those at the dinner remembered the poignancy with which Wells added, 'I hate the thought of leaving ... Few of my games are nearly finished and some I feel I have hardly begun.'

19

Settling Scores

Most obituaries written before the twentieth century were composed in the spirit of the Latin tag *De mortuis nil nisi bonum*, which can be loosely and colloquially translated as: only speak of the dead if you have something good to say. The consequence was that they read like panegyric. In the perhaps special case of a 'deceased friend or beloved kinsman', Wordsworth defended the habit of only being complimentary about the dead by claiming that they should be seen 'as a tree through a tender haze or a luminous mist, that spiritualises and beautifies it'; and he met the charge of untruthfulness by insisting that what then resulted was 'truth hallowed by love, the joint offspring of the worth of the dead and the affections of the living' (a formulation subtler than it seems in that it recognizes the inability of one human being to be entirely objective about another). By 1930 the assault on the Wordsworthian approach, in which Lytton Strachey's *Eminent Victorians* played such a crucial role, was well under way. Towards the beginning of his obituary of Lawrence, J. C. Squire says that '*de mortuis* is the most preposterous of all proverbs, for only of the dead can we speak the whole truth'. He probably meant that the pattern of someone's life only becomes clear after their death, although he may also have had in mind that in England the law of libel applies only to the living.

Wordsworth wrote at a time when the 'good name' of both the dead and the living mattered more than it does now, and there was more concern for the feelings of those relatives and friends the dead leave behind. There was also more respect for death itself. How could a phenomenon which manifested itself so frequently, and in such frightening and unpredictable ways, not be respected, especially when its next victim might be oneself? That some of these feelings survive is suggested both by the continuing restraint of most obituaries and the shock John Osborne was able to cause when, in the second volume of his autobiography, he published his reflections on the death of his fourth wife, Jill Bennett. She had committed suicide but in notebook entries apparently made on the day after the announcement of her death, Osborne denied her even that privilege, claiming that she had meant to be rescued and that, in accidentally killing herself, she was 'merely perpetuating a common little deceit under the delusion it was an expression of "style", rather than the coarse posturing of an overheated housemaid'. From the standpoint of what he announces as his own more intimate knowledge, Osborne then contests all the favourable comments on his former wife made in the obituaries, accusing her, among several other, similar weaknesses, of making money 'her undisputed reason for living', always having hid her real age, and being an incompetent actress who recited lines like 'a puppy with a mouthful of lavatory paper'. After their separation he had been in the habit of sending notes to Jill Bennett in which he addressed her as Adolf, and his inclination to pursue his antagonism beyond the grave is made especially evident in his response to the news, which followed several months after her death, that she had left half a million pounds to the Battersea Dogs' Home. Jill Bennett had, he maintains, 'no love in her heart for people and only a little more for dogs … Her frigidity was almost total. She loathed men and pretended to love women, whom she hated even more. She was at ease only in the company of homosexuals, whom she also despised but whose narcissism matched her own.' One might think that anyone willing to print these thoughts had done enough to demonstrate his belief that the mere fact of death should not prevent people from expressing honestly what they feel; but Osborne concludes his chapter with: 'I have only one regret remaining now in this matter of Adolf. It is simply that I was unable to look down upon her coffin and, like that bird in the Book of Tobias, drop a large, good mess in her eye.' For some it will be the whiff of desecration which makes this shocking but for others no more than the absence of fair play. Attacks so violent seem wrong when the victim is in no position to answer back.

Many people in the 1930s harboured bitter grudges against Lawrence but there is no posthumous attack on him at all comparable with that of Osborne's on his former wife. Probably in those years an attack of that nature would have been impossible, or at least unpublishable. Yet revenge can take many forms and even arrive in the cloak of charity or loving kindness. Murry had declared that Lawrence was the most lovable man he had ever known but by April 1931, working at a suspiciously impressive speed, he had published a full-scale biography which was remarkably hostile. *Son of Woman* was the book's title and it was almost as much an affront to Lawrence's friends as the chapter in Osborne's autobiography must have been to those of Jill Bennett.

Murry presents Lawrence as a hopelessly pathological case, such a victim of mother-love that he was 'incapable of loving a woman' and could never have satisfactory sexual relations. The entanglement of erotic feelings in his devotion to his mother meant that there was in his nature an 'irreparable inward division' between the spiritual and the physical. Since he was a man possessed of an 'extraordinary spiritual sensitiveness' but 'less than normal sexual vitality', he ought to have chosen to become a spiritual leader like Jesus but instead he willed himself into animality. Nature or nurture had made him 'almost a sexual weakling' so that the consequence of his going to women was that he failed to satisfy them, and did not the record show that he was unable to give them children? This failure on his part gave rise to a 'seething and bitter hatred' of women and, in his unavailing efforts to shake off his dependence on them, he attempted to establish several homosexual relations, but with no greater success than he enjoyed in the heterosexual sphere. According to Murry, Lawrence was a man who was 'doomed to spend his life distraught between humiliation and extravagant masculine assertion', who was mired in self-deception and 'adept at cheating himself with words', and the course of whose life was nothing more than a 'bitter tragedy'.

Son of Woman is not only long and detailed but also sufficiently clever to have been described by T. S. Eliot as 'brilliant' in a review he published in his journal the *Criterion*. It is written by someone with an unusually sharp eye for its subject's weaknesses; as Eliot said, here was a case where the victim and the sacrificial knife were perfectly adapted to each other. Murry is very familiar with Lawrence's writings and knows exactly where to go for a damaging quotation. He lays heavy stress on the chapter in *Sons and Lovers* in which, after persuading Miriam to sleep with him, Paul Morel then declares himself dissatisfied with the result. This is called in the novel 'The Test on Miriam' but Murry insists that, insofar as there is a test, it is not the woman who has failed it but the man. He draws attention to the more homoerotic passages in Lawrence's fiction: the scene in *The White Peacock* where one man dries the body of another after bathing; the famous naked wrestling in *Women in Love*; and more particularly, since it was very loosely based on his own experience with Lawrence, an episode in *Aaron's Rod* where a male character called Lilly massages with oil the naked body of the sick protagonist of the title. But his prize exhibit is Mellors's account of the women he has known in chapter 14 of *Lady Chatterley's Lover*, a novel he describes as 'wearisome and oppressive'. Murry assumes, and it has been widely accepted since, that the model for Mellors's description of 'the first girl (he) had', the one who stimulated his intellectual development but was unable to respond to him as a sexual being, must be Jessie Chambers. He feels he knows, and again later commentators have concurred, that the model for the woman who comes second on Mellors's list and who 'loved everything about love, except the sex', was Helen Corke, a teacher whom Lawrence had got to know in Croydon. But he realizes that this strongly suggests there must have been a real-life model for Mellors's third woman, Bertha Coutts (that there is no possible equivalent of Louie Burrows in the gamekeeper's list may suggest how guilty Lawrence continued to feel about her or only confirm that their year-long engagement had been comparatively unphysical). Bertha is described as always wanting to take the initiative in sexual intercourse so that she would wait until Mellors ejaculated and then bring herself off, 'grinding her own coffee'. 'By God,' he complains, 'you think a woman's soft down there, like a fig. But I tell you the old rampers have beaks between their legs, and they tear at you with it till you're sick. Self! Self! Self! all self! tearing and shouting! They talk about man's selfishness, but I doubt if it can ever touch a woman's blind beakishness, once she's gone that way.' These were startling phrases which in 1931 Murry was not able to quote in his book, but he describes their general tenor and makes it clear enough that in his view they could only refer to Lawrence's own experiences with his wife. He may have felt he was softening the blow for Frieda by asserting that what they obviously implied was not that her appetite for sex was voracious but that, even before he had become impotent, her husband had been sexually inadequate.

Frieda was not at all pacified. After *Son of Woman* was published she is said to have ceremoniously burnt her copy of the book so that she could post the ashes back to its author, and she took to reporting widely that Lawrence had been something of a sexual athlete in their first years together. What she also did was send a furious letter to Murry in which she accused him of having written *Son of Woman* for money. All she then had back were expressions of love more fervent than any he had ever sent her before. This must have seemed characteristic of the man who, while blackening the name of his former friend, simultaneously declared how much he loved, admired, and respected him. According to *Son of Woman*, Lawrence had many qualities which had made him comparable to Jesus, a biography of whom Murry had recently published; and was indeed Jesus-like in that he suffered for our sakes: 'he was a leader after the fashion of the man who leads because he suffers, who leads because he is crucified.' Although he was abnormal, 'it is the abnormal men from whom we have to learn . . . vital issues were tried to a conclusion in him'. The readers of *Son of Woman* must not therefore think that Murry is making any pretence of *judging* Lawrence (heaven forbid that he should dare to do so): 'One accepts him; he is what he is, a beautiful, suffering, divided, tormented being, driven by destiny to deny his own most wonderful faculties.' 'I hate "understanding" people', Lawrence had once said, adding that he hated still more 'to be understood', and he often expressed a particular fear of the 'understanding' woman. He could not know how, after his death, he would be in even more danger from the understanding man.

Admirers of Lawrence found Murry's tone objectionable but the more informed of them must also have been disgusted by the claim he made in the preface to the 1932 edition of his book that it was only in the writings that he had found the key to his subject, and that he had benefited from 'no backstairs knowledge, no secret information'. His book was in fact full of references to crucial moments in his long friendship with that subject and it was well known, in the appropriate literary circles, that he had both read an account which Jessie Chambers had already written of her relationship with Lawrence and (more importantly) slept with Frieda. This gave him advantages which many felt he had used unfairly and suggested that, if as he insisted Lawrence was indeed like Jesus, he had cast himself in the role of Judas. The familiar comparison with Jesus was one Lawrence himself had sometimes encouraged, wondering on one occasion why he had been sent to his 'cursed, rotten-boned, pappy-hearted countryman' and then adding: 'Christ on the cross must have hated his countrymen. "Crucify me you swine", he must have said through his teeth'; or more casually remarking at another time that the outbreak of the First World War had been like a spear through the side of all his hopes and aspirations. Yet he was capable of critical distance and gave a good deal of thought to an analysis of the leader/follower relationship, finally concluding that it was the fate of someone like Jesus not merely to attract figures like Judas, but also *deserve* them.

Murry was unusual in being able to indulge in reprehensible moral acts and always feel that he emerged smelling of roses. He gave himself the highest possible motives for writing *Son of Woman* but it was widely perceived as revenge for the way that, in his dealings with Lawrence, he had so often been in what he himself calls 'the subaltern position', or for the manner in which he had often been depicted in Lawrence's stories. When *Point Counter Point* was published, with a portrait of Murry as Burlap far more vicious than anything in Lawrence's work, he had claimed to be unaffected. Huxley has only 'rather beautifully confirmed', Murry wrote, 'my own strong impression that he hasn't very much notion of what I *am* driving at'. On only one occasion, he went on, had he been hurt and made to squirm by an attack of the kind Burlap represented, and this was when he read a short story by Lawrence. The difference was that he had 'a pretty deep admiration' for Lawrence which he did not feel for Huxley. 'In other terms', he concluded, 'DHL can stick the barb in deep, and AH can't.' Lawrence had often stuck the barb in deep and Murry was unlikely to have forgotten that when he had become editor of the *Athenaeum* just after the war, and solicited but then rejected a number of Lawrence's pieces, their author had called him a dirty little worm. It was their previous closeness which must have made insults of this kind hard to forget. As in the case of John Osborne and Jill Bennett, there is a settling of scores made more intense by a previous intimacy, certain kinds of betrayal of which only intimates are capable. When after his first stay in America, Lawrence came back to London at the end of 1923, he gave a dinner at the Café Royal for half a dozen of his closest friends. The intention was to see how many of them would be prepared to return with him to Taos and begin a new life there (Dorothy Brett and Murry both said they would but only Brett followed through). Too much wine was drunk and at one point Murry kissed Lawrence who is reported as having then asked him not to betray him. The others would have interpreted this remark as a reference to Frieda's recent trip with Murry to Germany but he himself later claimed that what he was being asked not to betray was his exclusive knowledge that Lawrence was no longer committed to 'life' but to death and despair. In the final two paragraphs of *Son of Woman* Murry reverts to the topic and, addressing his subject directly, admits that in his book he has betrayed Lawrence but then 'this "betrayal" was the one thing you lacked, the one thing I had to give'. Without it how could the world know that 'you were a man of destiny, driven to sacrifice yourself in order that men might know themselves?' From logic as twisted as this, Lawrence could only have turned away in despair. In 1929 he was offered a temptingly large sum of hush money by a rogue publisher who wanted him to endorse, retrospectively, a pirated edition of *Lady Chatterley's Lover*. Trying to explain why he felt he could not take it, Lawrence wrote: 'It is understood that

Judas is always ready with a kiss. But that I should have to kiss him back——!' Murry once claimed that Judas 'was the only one of the disciples to understand Jesus', but if he therefore imagined that Lawrence would have been grateful to have been 'betrayed', and prepared to kiss his own Judas back, he was surely mistaken.

20

Celebrations

I f it is foolish to speculate about how Lawrence would have responded to *Son of Woman*, the type of foolishness involved is very common. As the behaviour of Ada and Frieda demonstrates, imagining what the feelings of the dead would have been forms an important part of daily living. When supporting actors die in the middle of a run, the show goes on because 'that is what they would have wanted'. It is doubtful whether Murry could have written his book with the energy he did, had he not been able to imagine Lawrence as one of its readers. To tell him he was wasting his time would have been as useful as conveying the same message to tribesmen who were mutilating the corpses of their enemies.

The response Murry needed he could no doubt hypothesize but a rational approach to its reconstruction would be to ask how Lawrence responded to hostile commentary while he was still alive. If for a long time the sole reader of all he wrote was Jessie Chambers, it was because his exceptional self-consciousness as a young man meant that he feared public exposure and she represented the outside world at its most sympathetic. When at the beginning of 1912 he sent parts of his second novel, *The Trespasser*, to a friend, he said 'it is so much oneself, one's naked self. I give myself away too much, and write what is my most palpitant, sensitive self, that I loathe the book, because it will betray me to a parcel of fools'; and he went on to suggest that Stendhal must have writhed in torture every time he remembered that *Le Rouge et le noir* was public property. The critical reception of Lawrence's early books was in fact largely favourable and it was only when *The Rainbow* was banned by the authorities in 1915 that he began to suffer abuse. From then on he was often attacked in the press and became hardened to hostile criticism although he was never indifferent to it, as is illustrated by the episode in Port Cros when reviews of *Lady Chatterley's Lover* were read aloud. He had said then that 'Nobody *likes* being called a cesspool' and it is a safe bet that he would have been no exception to the rule that nobody *likes* being called 'almost a sexual weakling' either.

After *The Rainbow* had been banned, the prospects for Lawrence ever being able to publish its successor *Women in Love* became bleak. Yet he refused to give in, saying that if he went on writing it was 'to the unseen witnesses'. Every writer needs some kind of public but Lawrence was a man of exceptionally strong self-belief who was convinced that one day his voice would be heard and appreciated. When he was in New Mexico he was interviewed by a journalist who asked him why he wrote. Before he had time to answer Frieda intervened to say that his real motive was egotism and the desire to let everyone know how clever he was; but Lawrence then protested that on the contrary he wrote 'from a deep moral sense, for the race as it were'. The tenor of his remarks suggested how far he was an author in the nineteenth-century mould who believed in the mission of literature to change the world. 'I do write because I want folks to alter and have more sense,' he once declared. He was confident that if what he had to say was not especially well received immediately, it would come into its own later, even if that had to be after his death. Like Stendhal, he had faith in the future, if not in his contemporaries.

Stendhal died in 1842 and had been fond of suggesting that he would be read with enthusiastic understanding in 1880, a prediction which proved remarkably accurate. In spite of Murry, posterity did not let Lawrence down either, even in the years which immediately followed his death. Most of the many books or pamphlets which then appeared were celebratory. An important boost to his reputation was provided by the publication in 1932 of more than eight hundred pages of his letters. (The refusal of both Enid Hilton and Aldous Huxley to accept payment for their work in collecting and editing these meant a large advance for Frieda, which may have been a factor in her decision to pay off George and Emily.) In the introduction to the volume, Huxley began by describing *Son of Woman* as a 'curious essay in destructive hagiography' and then made the dubious claim that, if Lawrence's mother had died when he was a child, he 'would still have been, essentially and fundamentally, Lawrence' (in private he had said that Murry's book represented 'the slug's-eye view' of its subject). He went on to convey a warm and highly favourable impression of his dead friend which, influential though it became, was to prove less important than the letters themselves. They offered a volatile mixture of passion, wit, vivid description, and psychological insight whose equivalent could only be found in the letters of Keats or Byron. It was often said of Byron that his fame depended as much on the force of his personality as on his writing. Something similar would also be said of Lawrence. Yet although it was through biographies or memoirs that the public became aware of Lawrence's personality, it was conveyed most directly through his letters, many of which contain 'writing' of the highest order.

The appetite in England for more details of Lawrence meant that in 1931 Ada was able to publish her *Young Lorenzo*, a memoir of his early life together with letters and reproductions of his early paintings. In the following year Catherine Carswell replied to *Son of Woman* with a wholly favourable portrait of Lawrence in her biography, *The Savage Pilgrimage*, making in the process a series of scornful, disparaging references to the way Murry had treated Lawrence while he was still alive. The dead may not be able to sue for libel but the living certainly can and Carswell was forced by Murry to withdraw her book although she soon found another publisher willing to print a slightly modified version. In 1933 Murry collected together a number of *Reminiscences of D. H. Lawrence* which had previously appeared in his *Adelphi* magazine and seized the opportunity to write a point-by-point rebuttal of all Carswell's criticisms of his behaviour. In the preface to this volume he insisted that the part he had been called on to play in Lawrence's life 'was that of the friend who understood' and that, although he had failed to answer the call during Lawrence's lifetime, he had been able to do so after his death. The vast majority of Lawrence's other friends felt that he ought not to have bothered and the Brewsters were among them. In 1934 they published a volume which was also called *Reminiscences* and which, although it certainly showed that Lawrence could be idiosyncratic and unpredictable, presented him as in the main warmly sympathetic, energizing, wise, and the obverse of neurotic.

The degree of American interest in Lawrence after his death was comparable to that in Britain and the most important, immediate responses to it came from three women who were all then living in or around Taos. Each of them had wanted him for herself but in only one had the want been satisfied. When Mabel Luhan first invited Lawrence to Taos it was in the hope that he would be a powerful aid in her campaign to help the American Indian, but once he was there she also decided that Frieda was no longer a suitable partner for him. 'You *need* something new and different,' she told him, 'You have done her. She has mothered your books long enough. You need a new mother,' and she proposed herself for the role. Lawrence declined her offer and did not always write about the American Indian in quite the way she wanted. This helped to make *Lorenzo in Taos*, the memoir Mabel published in 1932, less positive than it might have been; but the portrait she paints is nevertheless a sympathetic one. If it now seems slightly disapproving it is perhaps in comparison with Dorothy Brett's *Lawrence and Brett: A Friendship* which appeared the next year. The tone of this book makes its subtitle a classic instance of British understatement since it everywhere reveals that Brett (as she was always called) worshipped Lawrence. When she and the Lawrences established an uneasy *ménage à trois* in Mexico in 1924, an exasperated Frieda accused her and Lawrence of being like a curate and a spinster and suggested that their relationship would be less unhealthy if they did have sex together. Their failed attempt to take up this suggestion in Capri in 1926 left Frieda again triumphant as she had previously been over Mabel.

Frieda admitted that were she to describe all the difficulties of living with Lawrence the result would 'not be a pretty book but rather terrible'. '*Not I, but the wind . . .* ' is the title of the memoir she published in 1934 and in it she rejected that approach and produced instead a lively and often moving celebration of her marriage. In 1913, while she was still not yet divorced but living with Lawrence in Italy, he had written to Jessie Chambers and somewhat insensitively admitted that he and Frieda discussed her endlessly. Jessie fantasized that Frieda's contribution to the discussion would consist of assurances of 'Miriam's fundamental unsuitability for the job of life-partner to D.H.L.' and her own intrinsic aptitude. '*Not I, but the wind . . .* ' was among many other things an affirmation of that intrinsic aptitude but then, with all her competitors routed, history appeared to be firmly on her side. Jessie was later reduced to claiming that it was only 'in eternity' that she would always figure as Frieda's symbolic opposite, the option Lawrence could and should have taken.

D. H. Lawrence: A Personal Record, the memoir in which Jessie Chambers denied the 'fundamental unsuitability' of Miriam as Lawrence's life partner, did not appear until 1935. This is surprising given that she had always had literary aspirations. Shortly after the break with Lawrence, she completed a novel based on her early experience, which she eventually called *Eunice Temple* ('E.T.' was the pseudonym she adopted for *A Personal Record*). While it was being considered for publication, David Garnett's father, Edward, sent a copy to Lawrence who said that it was not bad but also that the matters with which it dealt had made him so miserably unhappy that he had hardly had the energy to walk out of the house for two days. The novel did not appear and Jessie later burnt the manuscript but by the end of 1930 she clearly had an autobiographical account of her relations with Lawrence which Murry was able to read. By then Lawrence's death had brought her unwelcome publicity. In his own 'Autobiographical Sketch' he had described how Jessie had sent some of his poems to the *English Review* and thereby launched his literary career, 'like a princess cutting a thread, launching a ship'. In April 1930 *The Star* newspaper published a long 'Talk with Lawrence's "Princess"' in which their journalist managed to wring from Jessie the belief that Lawrence's life had been a tragedy and that 'his last writings and those terrible paintings ought never to have been given to the world'. Catching her between spring-cleaning and the preparation of her husband's midday meal (she had married a schoolteacher in 1915), he was also able to report her murmuring, as she looked at a pocket set of Hardy, 'If only he had written books like those'. The interview makes clear that Jessie was unhappy with the attention which had come her way, as was also Louie Burrows. But her situation became much more uncomfortable than Louie's when in the following year Murry's book appeared with its heavy stress on her sexual relationship with Lawrence. If she held back from telling her side of the story, it may have been because she preferred to wait until the spotlight had become less glaring.

There is nothing in *A Personal Record* to indicate that its author and Lawrence ever slept together but this important omission does not prevent it from being an excellent book. Jessie celebrates the golden age of her and Lawrence's youth and in the process gives the lie to those who, like Squire or T. S. Eliot, were inclined to suggest that his shortcomings could largely be attributed to a culturally deprived social background. She shows how lively the intellectual life centred on the Congregationalist chapel in Eastwood could be, and how well read she and Lawrence managed to become, in French as well as in English literature. What she conveys particularly well is the almost sensuous thrill of living in a world of continually widening intellectual and artistic horizons. The prose in which she writes is mostly expository, lucid, and sober, but there are occasional moments of effective dramatization. One of these comes in her description of the period when she was 19 and Lawrence 20. They had just enjoyed an exceptionally happy time together and Lawrence had promised to call on her the next day in the early afternoon. But it was late when he did arrive and his mood had altered. It turned out that on the previous evening his sister Emily had asked his mother whether he and Jessie were courting, and that the two women had then explained that he would be compromising Jessie by being so often alone in her company unless he decided he wanted to become engaged. But he had looked into his heart and could not find that he loved her 'as a husband should love his wife'.

This was the watershed in Jessie's relations with Lawrence. The way she interprets it in retrospect is to insist that it was Mrs Lawrence who prevented her son from having proper feelings for her, or indeed for any other woman. Her final analysis of arrested development is very close to Murry's, who may well have borrowed parts of it from her. *A Personal Record* is therefore in one sense a celebration but in another a damning judgement. In passing that judgement Jessie cannot admit that there was ever anything inadequate about herself, or that she was simply not the kind of woman to whom Lawrence could be physically attracted. After his sister and mother had spoken to him, he perhaps made an error in insisting that he valued Jessie too much as a friend and literary confidant to give her up; and he was certainly wrong to have persuaded her later into having sex with him on the grounds that he may have been mistaken about his previous feelings. But Jessie could also have broken the relationship off, or at least said no to his persuasions. If she did not do either it was because she loved Lawrence deeply, but also because she could never stop believing that they were soul-mates, and that, whatever he and other people might say, she was the only right person for him.

The arrival of the proofs of *Sons and Lovers*, together with the fact that Lawrence was now living abroad with Frieda, finally persuaded Jessie to cut off all communications by sending back his letter. This allowed him to suggest that 'she was bitterly ashamed of having had me, as if I had dragged her spiritual plumage in the mud'; but at the same time he admitted that 'it hurt when she sent a letter of mine back'. Before taking that decisive step, Jessie had strengthened her resolve by remembering that Lawrence had once said to her, 'An ounce of justice is worth a ton of generosity. Any woman will give a man a ton of generosity, but is there a woman who will give him an ounce of justice?' She says that as she sent back his letter she could not refrain from thinking, 'Here is your ounce of justice', and she would have no doubt applied these same words to the analysis of his problems which appears in *A Personal Record*.

It is clear that justice remained an important concept for Lawrence from his own, single attempt at a biographical memoir, the long introduction to Maurice Magnus's *Memoirs of the French Foreign Legion*. It was in 1920 that Magnus had sought Lawrence out in Sicily in order to borrow some money. On several occasions he was successful but eventually strong prompting from Frieda made Lawrence feel that he must refuse any further help. The relationship of the two men nevertheless continued a brief while longer after Magnus had retreated to Malta, Lawrence happened to take a short holiday there, and two kind Maltese showed both of them round the island. Being in another country did not protect Magnus from those to whom he owed money and his suicide quickly followed. It was after hearing of his death that Lawrence arranged to have Magnus's memoirs published and to precede them with his own account of their author. His purpose was to earn at least enough money to recover what he had lent Magnus but also sufficient to pay back the two Maltese whom he had met in his company (having been persuaded into providing small loans they had appealed to Lawrence as to how they might be reimbursed). If he also wanted to work out the enigma of the dead man's strangely appealing and exasperating character, a further aim was perhaps to convince both himself and others that there was no reason to feel guilty for having helped to seal Magnus's fate by refusing to lend him any more money. Lawrence regarded his long memoir or introduction as the best writing, '*as writing*', that he had ever done and there is enough truth in his claim to make it a pity that only Lawrence specialists have ever heard of it. Its conclusion picks up the theme which Jessie evoked to explain her own actions to herself and includes the ringing assertion that 'the dead ask only for *justice*: not praise or exoneration. Who dares humiliate the dead with excuses for their living? . . . Forgiveness gives the whimpering dead no rest. Only deep, true justice.'

Lawrence would have known that in a godless world, or one inhabited by only his kind of gods, the call that the dead should have justice which was deep and true can never be fully answered because all justice of the human variety is partial. What he therefore must have meant is that when fellow humans judge the dead they should try as hard as they can to put aside all personal resentments or sympathies, to be as objective as possible. But Jessie would have said that she had done this, as would Middleton Murry. In 1951 a short memoir of Jessie Chambers was published by Helen Corke, the second on Mellors's list of the women who had mattered in his life. A common interest in Lawrence had led her and Jessie to become friends, and they had spent several happy holidays together. The last time they met was in 1940 but then Helen Corke could hardly recognize the bent, heavy figure who approached her. Jessie explained that she was recovering from a nervous breakdown which had left her deaf and as she began to talk 'with smouldering resentment, of the war, of her illness, of the shabby treatment of the book, which had been printed in an American edition without her sanction'. All Helen Corke could feel was pity. Jessie sensed this and, turning her resentment against her former friend, 'rose to go, averting her face'. The spectacle of collapse Helen Corke presents is a harrowing one, powerfully evoked, but how would it be possible to estimate the degree of deep justice there would be in holding Lawrence wholly or at least partly responsible for having brought it about?

21

Mortal Remains

Frieda revelled in her status as the widow of a great writer: it brought her the attention she felt she deserved. 'Do you know how much liberating I did for Lawrence,' she wrote to Brett after his death, 'It was given to me to make him flower.' When Ada criticized her for putting on airs, she was unaware of the notions of a woman's mission in life which Frieda had imbibed from elements in her German culture, and particularly from the affair she had with a highly unorthodox psychoanalyst called Otto Gross while she was still married to Weekley. What these had suggested to her was that by uniting herself to a man of potential genius, a strong-willed woman could still make her mark in a male-dominated world. The model was not the old one of the humble helpmate who liberates her more creative partner from material concerns by taking care of those household chores which (as it happens) largely became Lawrence's province when he and Frieda lived together, but rather of the vibrant female whose erotic power both energizes and clarifies the mind of the male. This was woman not as useful adjunct but as indispensable resource and stimulation, and the art which resulted therefore belonged as much to her as to her partner. During the first years of living with Frieda, Lawrence accepted this view of their relationship, saying, for example, that *Sons and Lovers* was the work of both of them and telling a friend in 1914 that he thought the only way to revivify art was to make it more the joint work of man and woman. Later, and especially in what is known as the 'leadership' phase of his writing, he tried to persuade Frieda that, as his wife, she ought to adopt a more subservient role. But subservience was not in her nature and, once she was his widow, it was to those early years when he had acknowledged her importance and power that her mind returned.

Enjoying the limelight as she did, it may seem strange that Frieda was willing to go back to Taos, but the ranch was the only property she owned and she was very attached to it. Ada was never her greatest fan but admitted that she admired Frieda for having endured Lawrence's disinclination to settle and for being willing to follow him round the world. The ranch was now her home and she relished the daily routine of living there. Although it was Lawrence who for most of their marriage had made the fires, scrubbed the floors, and brought her breakfast in bed, Frieda did have a domestic side and loved to bake. Once described by Otto Gross as a woman of the future whose laughter and loving had kept her soul free of 'the curse and dirt of two gloomy millennia', she was also fond of needlework and knitting. On the ranch, with its beautiful surroundings and spectacular view way down to the fissure on the sage-brush plain which hid the Rio Grande, she could indulge her talent for happy pottering, or happily doing nothing, which Lawrence had so appreciated. When Mabel Luhan was in town there would be plenty of interesting people to meet and one important advantage of Taos was that it was a largely artistic, bohemian community. Living there with someone else's husband twelve years younger than oneself presented none of the problems which might have arisen in very many other, more conventional locations.

Already being married was one of the drawbacks of Angelo and according to Barby, who never liked him, another was that he was not very bright. In an interview he gave towards the end of his life he said that he had tried to read *Sons and Lovers* but found it too heavy, '*much* too heavy. We don't need literature to know what to do.' He had been wounded and decorated during the First World War and when he first arrived in Taos was a fervent supporter of Mussolini. This cannot have made things easier after Pearl Harbor when he became an enemy alien, as indeed did Frieda, but influential friends seem to have helped them both to remain unmolested. Perhaps his political views became more moderate with time, but that was not true of his womanizing. An American who knew him in the 1940s said that he 'screwed anything he could'. As Frieda moved into her middle and late sixties she became reconciled to giving him a comparatively free rein even though, throughout their time together, he represented a considerable drain on her resources. Although Angelo eventually turned his hand to pottery and managed to sell some pieces, it was Frieda (or rather Lawrence through Frieda) who was always the breadwinner. She supported not only Angelo but also his wife and children since she supplemented to a limited extent his army pension which it had already been agreed they should receive. In 1950 Frieda decided that everything would be simpler if she and Angelo married: it would be easier then for him to apply for an American passport which would allow him to travel abroad without any anxiety about not being allowed to return to her. With what must have been his wife's reluctant approval, Angelo secured a divorce in Las Vegas. This was satisfactory to the authorities in America but not to those in Italy so that when, after Frieda's death, he returned to Italy his status had not changed and he could resume his old life as a husband and father. With half the proceeds of Frieda's estate he must then have seemed to outsiders like many other Italians who returned home from the United States having made good or, with the Lawrence boom in the 1960s and 1970s, very good indeed.

Circumstances tend to make Angelo look bad but, with the exception of Barby, Frieda's friends and relatives liked him. The Huxleys, who were good judges, thought that he looked after Frieda well and was genuinely solicitous for her welfare. Intensely practical, he worked hard on building the new house on the ranch and repairing or renovating the properties Frieda bought nearer to Taos and on the Gulf of Mexico. If he had been no more than a vulgar adventurer she would not have continued the arrangement for so long, or married him in 1950. They got on well but although what became known as the 'upper' ranch was isolated, and the road to it sometimes impassable in winter, she was not limited to his company even there. A steady stream of young admirers made their way to see both the woman who had shared her life with Lawrence and an environment he had described so vividly in stories like 'St. Mawr'. A short, dumpy figure in old age who liked to wear brightly patterned Native American clothing, and the remnants of whose former beauty could be found in a fine profile and arresting green eyes, Frieda became over the years the priestess of a cult; and yet no one could be less mysterious or hieratic. Warm, welcoming, and voluble she would entertain her visitors with home baking, anecdotes of the literary celebrities she and Lawrence had known (told in what was still a strong German accent), and instances of his remarkable understanding and insight.

Every cult needs a shrine at which its followers can worship. From the moment of Lawrence's death Frieda had wanted to bring his body to New Mexico and on her return to the ranch she had quickly identified a rise above the old cabin which would be suitable for a small mausoleum or temple. But she was deterred by the likely expense. In 1934 an article appeared in a French journal which described how ill-kept Lawrence's grave was, and the general poor state of the Vence cemetery. This angered a local official who wrote a letter claiming that it was only the good nature of the municipality which prevented Lawrence's body from being dug up and placed in common ground because his plot had never been paid for. Prompted by Martha Crotch (who is the source of this information), Huxley replied with a formal denial. The dispute attracted worldwide publicity and led Frieda to tell Angelo that on his coming trip back home to see his family he should go to Vence, have Lawrence's body exhumed and cremated, and then bring the ashes back to her.

This was a complicated operation and Earl Brewster was heavily involved in all the paperwork required. In Vence itself Frieda was able to count on the help of her good friend Martha Crotch, who was the person to whom visitors were always directed when they wanted to see Lawrence's grave. She had been born Martha Gordon in Hartlepool and it was only in 1929 that she became Crotch by deed poll in what must now seem to outsiders an exceptional gesture of affection for a journalist with that unappealing name who worked in the area. Well known in the local artistic and literary circles, she had been able to introduce Frieda to Emma Goldman, and to the widow of Frank Harris, the writer whose scandalous autobiography, *My Life and Loves*, had caught Lawrence's interest just before he began to write *Lady Chatterley's Lover*. But meeting Frieda's friends further enriched her life and she became so attached to Norman Douglas that, when he had to leave Italy in 1937 for alleged interference with a minor, she sheltered him in her house in Vence. The appropriateness here is that whereas Douglas was universally known as 'uncle' Martha Crotch was always referred to by her friends as 'auntie'. A loyal but also (her writings suggest) a sensible friend, she was essential to Angelo if he wanted to complete the difficult job Frieda had given him.

Following a request made to the local authorities by Martha Crotch on Frieda's behalf, the exhumation of Lawrence's body was fixed for 12 March 1935. Angelo arrived the day before, bringing news of Taos and expressing anxiety about securing the visa he would need to return there. Early next morning Martha Crotch went to the cemetery to find the exhumation almost completed. There was a small zinc-lined casket in which 'all that remained of poor Lorenzo was being placed'. It did not amount to much, 'just a few spadefuls of unrecognisable matter, but among it a hairbrush appeared intact and horribly fresh looking'. She was given photographs which recorded the moment the coffin was opened and which showed that, although the body had then been in a decent state of preservation, it quickly crumbled to dust once exposed to the air. The most famous account of the exhumation of a writer's body is in Trelawny's *Recollections of the last days of Byron and Shelley*, a book Lawrence knew well. Shelley had drowned in the Gulf of Spezia but his recovered body had been buried on shore and Trelawny obtained permission to disinter it. The skull, he noted, had turned a 'dark and ghastly indigo colour' because of the lime which had been used in the burial. In a portable furnace he had brought with him, Trelawny was allowed to cremate Shelley's remains on the spot and records that, as the front of the skull fell off, the brains 'seethed and bubbled' in the hollow part which remained; and that he burnt his hand snatching the heart from the fire after he noticed that it had 'remained entire'. These are gruesome details but they do make the episode memorable and give it a certain Romantic glamour. They make it an occasion. In Martha Crotch's account, Lawrence's exhumation, most of which she missed, is not an occasion. Angelo missed it altogether. By the time he arrived, complaining that the people at his hotel had failed to wake him up, the casket had been sealed. He accompanied it in a hearse to Marseilles; it was delivered to the crematorium there at nine o'clock the next day; and the ashes were ready for collection at ten thirty, 'after cooling'.

Reliable knowledge of what happened afterwards is chiefly dependent on the Baron Prosper de Haulleville. He was the brother of a man who married Maria Huxley's sister Rose and it was with Rose (then widowed) that he visited the Taos ranch after Frieda's death. Angelo was at that time preparing to return to Italy, full of anxieties as to how his wife and family would receive him but, more particularly, about whether he would be accepted back into the Catholic Church. In two long, Bourbon-fuelled conversations he confessed his sins. He was remorseful about having been unfaithful to Frieda as well as his wife, and feared that the Church would not approve of what he called, in the French he appears to have spoken well, 'l'argent de la stupre' (money earned from debauchery). 'Is it honest for my *true* wife and children to become rich because of their husband and father's guilt?', he asked. He regretted that he had painted a number of erotic pictures which he was able to sell more easily by falsely ascribing them to Frieda, but his chief confession concerned Lawrence's ashes. He said that in order to avoid complications he had left these in Marseilles and filled an appropriate urn with substitute material once he was back in New York. Those who met de Haulleville later described him as entirely trustworthy and it is hard to see what purpose Angelo could have had in telling him a story which was not true.

In addition to '*Not I, but the wind . . .* ', Frieda wrote parts of a fictionalized autobiography never published during her lifetime. In this work she describes how grateful she felt that 'Dario' (as she calls Angelo) 'had a respect almost as her own' for Lawrence's memory. She says that when he returned from Europe with the ashes and she met him at the station in Lamy, close to Santa Fe, he was 'very quiet' because 'he was like that when he was moved'. But perhaps Angelo was quiet because he was feeling apprehensive and guilty. Frieda was in any event so pleased to see him that she drove off leaving the ashes behind and then had to double back to Lamy in order to retrieve them. Once in Taos she showed a pride in their possession which seems to have irritated Brett and Mabel. They talked of stealing the precious urn and scattering the ashes in the countryside Lawrence had found so impressive and invigorating. Before leaving for Europe, Angelo had already built the adobe temple where Frieda kept the urn (Brett thought it looked like a station toilet), but now she made the supposed ashes safe by having them mixed with the concrete which provided this construction with an altar.

'Who knows the fate of his bones, or how often he is to be buried?, asks Sir Thomas Browne at the beginning of *Urne-Burial*, 'who hath the oracle of his ashes, or whither they are to be scattered?' Like Lawrence, the great seventeenth-century letter writer Madame de Sévigné was also buried quietly in Provence but during the French Revolution her body was disinterred and a local lawyer had one of her teeth set in a ring as if it were a precious stone. If the dead have very little control over the image which survives them, they have scarcely any more over what happens to their mortal remains, even when those remains are genuine. Frieda could have dedicated her temple to Lawrence without the bother of the ashes but she was motivated by the same feelings which led Trelawny to take Shelley's remains to Rome for burial or caused the Greeks to insist on keeping Byron's lungs before his body was shipped back to England. There are obvious analogies in these famous cases with the relics of the Saints of which it is often said that there are many more of the former than there were of the latter, just as the surviving remnants of the true cross would make up far more than one. But belief is what counts and that strange, irrational difference many feel between a monument which only calls on us to think of the dead and one which also claims to harbour their remains. Melville makes the distinction in his characteristically florid way when in *Moby Dick* Ishmael is standing in a chapel among women who have lost their sailor loved ones at sea: 'Oh! ye whose dead lie buried beneath the green grass; who standing among flowers can say—here, *here* lies my beloved, ye know not the desolation that broods in bosoms like these. What bitter blanks in those black-bordered marbles which cover no ashes!' On a quite different level is the anxiety recently expressed by the Anglican Church about parishioners who, having obtained permission to bury their loved ones in their gardens, then move to other parts of the country and insist on taking the disinterred remains with them.

One of Frieda's role models while Lawrence was still alive could well have been her exact contemporary Alma Schindler. She was married to Gustav Mahler and, after his death, had a tempestuous affair with Oskar Kokoschka who told her, 'I must have you for my wife soon, or else my great talent will perish miserably. You must revive me at night like a magic potion.' Once Lawrence was dead and beyond revival, Frieda could no longer be his erotic muse and so became instead the keeper of his flame. For that role the world of German culture offered at least one prominent model from an earlier generation. Much to her brother's disgust, Elisabeth Nietzsche married a rabid anti-Semite who took her to Paraguay, away from 'international Jewry', in order to found an Aryan colony. When this ran into difficulties, and he committed suicide, she was forced to come back home. There she set about establishing control of the papers of her dear brother Fritz and freezing out those philosopher friends of his who might provide a challenge to her authority. Since his work was to represent not only her mission but also her future livelihood, she persuaded her mother to sign all rights over to her. With ruthless efficiency she supervised the various editors she employed to work on the many unpublished manuscripts, produced a considerably doctored official rather than authorized biography, and in general ensured that it was *her*

Nietzsche which the world should see. What is unusual about this process is that, for the first few years of it, Nietzsche was still alive, sitting in an adjoining room staring into space, emitting the occasional bellow, and being exhibited by Elisabeth to a few, highly privileged visitors (though he went mad in 1889 he did not die until 1900). The climax of her career can be seen in a famous photograph taken in 1933. This shows her outside the large and elegant building in Weimar which she had succeeded in acquiring in order to house the Nietzsche archives. A charming little old lady, she is extending a warm and smiling welcome to the recently appointed Reich Chancellor, Adolf Hitler, and symbolically delivering her brother's legacy into his hands. 'Fritz would have been enchanted by Hitler,' she is reported as saying. That Nietzsche had detested her husband is only one of the many reasons why her claim seems doubtful, but the truth is that Fritz died too soon for her or any of us to be certain what he would have felt.

No one person can control the legacy of any writer or thinker for long. No amount of suppression, of selective quotation, or of the kind of minor forgery Elisabeth Nietzsche sometimes practised will in the long run protect the work from rival interpretations. Frieda may have instinctively known this but she was in any case far more easy-going than Nietzsche's fearsome sister. Thinking of Lawrence's friends in her fictionalized autobiography, she wrote 'It had not been given to them to understand him, not one'. The implication is obvious but, though she knew what she knew, she was tolerant of the mistakes friends made. When she took her first visit to Taos after Lawrence's death, Mabel showed her the typescript of *Lorenzo in Taos*. Although Frieda disliked it and thought it gave a false impression of Lawrence, she did not insist on any changes as Mabel had feared she might. Detesting *Son of Woman* did not prevent her from collaborating with Murry in the matter of the will or maintaining a warm relationship with him afterwards. People were clearly, in her opinion, free to think what mistaken thoughts they liked. A friend like Huxley felt she had a simplified view of Lawrence's meaning and message, one that reflected her own straightforward nature rather than her husband's highly complicated one. At one point in his novel *Point Counter Point* he has the Lawrence figure interrupt his wife with 'Oh, for God's sake shut up'. When she then protests that what she has been saying is only what he himself often says, the figure replies with, 'What I say is what *I say*. It becomes different when you say it.' As an interpreter of Lawrence's work, Frieda may have had her limitations but as the keeper of his flame she had none of the desire Elisabeth Nietzsche showed to force her interpretations on the world.

22

Apotheosis

I n 1919 Max Beerbohm published an elegant and ingenious short story about literary fame. Its title is provided by the central character, Enoch Soames, who is imaginary although there are several historical figures with whom he is shown rubbing shoulders, including Beerbohm himself. Soames is a typical poet from the 1890s, outlandishly dressed, devoted to French literature, fond of absinthe, and often to be found at London's Café Royal now that he no longer lives in Paris. Contemptuous of all conventional moral standards, he declares himself to be a 'Catholic diabolist'. He has produced three slim volumes and tries to hide from others his despair at their failure to secure him any reasonable degree of attention. When Beerbohm meets him one day at lunchtime in a Soho restaurant, Soames confesses his frustration and admits that a great artist's faith in himself, and in the verdict of posterity, is not enough to keep him happy. 'Posterity!', he says, 'What use is it *to me*? A dead man doesn't know that people are visiting his grave—visiting his birthplace—putting up tablets to him—unveiling statues of him. A dead man can't read the books that are written about him.' Because he frequents the reading room of the British Museum (when he is not at the Café Royal), he declares that he would sell both his body and soul in order to be projected into that room as it will be in a hundred years' time, and he imagines all the satisfaction he would then feel in being able to read the numerous pages in the catalogue which he feels certain would be devoted to him. A gentleman of Mephistophelean aspect also present in the restaurant overhears these words and offers to take up the bargain they propose. After a brief negotiation Soames is whisked away into the future on the understanding that he will be back in the restaurant at dinner time so that the devil can collect his dues. Beerbohm makes sure that before this happens he himself is back at the restaurant to see Soames. This is in order to suggest what prove to be inevitably fruitless methods the poet might employ to escape the consequences of his Faustian pact, but also to satisfy a natural curiosity as to what the reading room had revealed. A downcast Soames explains that on the afternoon of 3 June 1997 there were no additions to his three items in the British Library catalogue, and that the only other sign of his having ever existed was a reference in a handbook on the literature of the 1890s to a short story by Max Beerbohm in which he had appeared.

If Lawrence had been able to visit the British Library in June 1997 he would have had the satisfaction Soames anticipated but was denied: 'think of the pages and pages... endless editions, commentaries, prolegomena, biographies...'. The quantity may have surprised him but he would certainly have been astonished by the group which had gathered in 1985, twelve years earlier, in order to unveil a stone to his memory in Westminster Abbey ('Think how many royal bones | Sleep within these heaps of stones', as Francis Beaumont put it in a poem from which Lawrence quotes in one of his letters). An uneasy combination of national mausoleum and house of Christian worship, the Abbey's imposing architecture is obscured and sometimes defaced by huge monuments to the dead from a grateful nation, the tombs of monarchs as well as other celebrated figures, and memorials to individuals now so anonymous that the visitor is bound to feel that they were able to exert undue influence, or had a lot of money. It is hard to imagine what the groups of foreign tourists who shuffle round can deduce from this mixture about the national scale of values. The principle of heterogeneity which operates in general is also relevant to that part of the Abbey known as 'poet's corner' whose occupants remind one of Addison's witty remark that although there are many poets without memorials, there are also many memorials without poets. According to Cecil Day Lewis, who in his then capacity of poet laureate introduced a guide to poet's corner in the early 1970s, its 'muddle' is only 'apparent' and its 'arbitrary and unplanned nature . . . one of its most rewarding features'. This was because 'the moralist may draw from it useful lessons about the transience of human reputations and the permanence of human values'. If what Day Lewis meant was that no one walking through what is now no longer a corner, and certainly not the exclusive preserve of poets, could fail to notice many names of writers no longer read, and the absence of even more who are now admired, then what he should perhaps have said is that, in a living culture where the list of admired writers is constantly being modified, any attempt to celebrate the finest of them will always over time risk appearing muddled, however systematic and organized the origins of that attempt may be.

Securing a berth or sign of recognition in poet's corner has always been something of a lottery and can often involve considerable delay. Lawrence had to wait fifty-five years for his stone to be unveiled, or a century if one begins counting from his birth. It was placed just below one commemorating Lord Byron, which was not laid until 1969. Although the Greeks insisted on keeping Byron's lungs as a *memento mori*, approaches were made to the Abbey's dignitaries about the burial there of the rest of his body when it was brought back to England in 1824, but they were firmly rejected. The points at issue presumably included his lordship's reputation for scandalous behaviour of a sexual nature and his attitude to Christianity, on both of which Lawrence might also have been found wanting. But by the 1980s Richard Hoggart had characterized Lawrence as a 'puritan' in the trial of *Lady Chatterley* while several other witnesses had spoken warmly of his monogamous nature; and although he had often attacked the Church of England and satirized its officials, he had always displayed a deep, well-informed interest in Christianity and could with justice be broadly described as religious. Not that this last attribute seems to have been particularly important to the Dean of Westminster who, in welcoming the congregation to the unveiling of Lawrence's stone, said only that it represented 'a tribute to a serious writer handling serious themes relating to our human predicament and man's fulfilment'.

Because there is an engraving of a phoenix on Lawrence's stone, it stands out from its neighbours in his particular cluster on the floor or pavement of poet's corner. He adopted this symbol during the war years when the attempt to rise from the ashes of an old life into a new had become a recurrent physical and psychological necessity. Thereafter the phoenix was closely associated with him, appearing on the cover of the Florence edition of *Lady Chatterley's Lover* as well as on his gravestone in Vence. When Frieda transferred what she believed were his remains to Taos, she made sure there was a phoenix symbol on the roof of the temple which Angelo built. In modern parlance the phoenix could accurately be described as Lawrence's logo and might suggest that he had an early, intuitive understanding of what is now called branding. There is a peculiarity about the way he chose to refer to himself which might support this suggestion. His first initial stands for David but he disliked the name and hardly ever used it. In a comic account in one of his essays, he describes how the headmaster of his elementary school would become purple with indignation at the irrationality of this dislike: 'You don't like the name of David! David is the name of a great and good man.' His second name of Herbert was always shortened to Bert so that during his childhood and adolescence he was 'our Bert' to all his family. After his sister Emily had been to visit him late in his life, he reflected sadly on the gulf between his interests and hers and said, 'I am not really "our Bert". Come to think of it, I never was.' A proof of this claim is that in his earliest letters and postcards he never signs himself either David or Bert but always D. H. Lawrence or DHL, and he maintained this habit later, even when he was writing to someone who meant as much to him as Louie Burrows. It is as if, modelling himself on well-known authors such as R. L. Stevenson or H. G. Wells, he had deliberately chosen the form of his name which he felt would go best with his phoenix logo well before it had been adopted by him, or he had published a single word.

This apparent concern with branding in the modern fashion did not protect Lawrence from being branded in a quite different sense. A feature of his work is its remarkable variety. He is not only the author of many of the twentieth century's most memorable depictions of English working-class life but also, in his major novels, of startlingly original depictions of the underground and barely definable feelings which occur in all intense relationships. A poet of distinction, he wrote many short stories and novellas which are as good as any in English literature, and also four excellent travel books. One or two of his plays are well worth seeing and in scores of essays and reviews, and several short books, he challenged his contemporaries' thinking on politics, art, psychology, or religion in what was always a highly distinctive but also, often, a peculiarly sharp and intelligent manner. Yet by the general public the only work for which Lawrence is now really remembered is *Lady Chatterley's Lover*: if he was ever successfully branded, it was above all as that novel's bearded author. This was made clear enough on the day following the unveiling of his stone when it was the *Sunday Times* and not a tabloid newspaper which ran the headline, '"Dirty Bertie" makes it to the Abbey'.

Lawrence's stone is distinguished from those in its vicinity not only by its phoenix but also by its epitaph or motto. Of his near neighbours only Byron has one of these: 'But there is that within me which shall tire | Torture and Time, and breathe when I expire.' The lines are from *Childe Harold's Pilgrimage* and express a sentiment familiar to most people from Shakespeare's sonnets. The words on Lawrence's stone read: '*Homo sum!* the Adventurer'. They are taken from an essay never published in his lifetime entitled 'Climbing down Pisgah' and, although they might remind some well-informed visitors of Lawrence's preference for the unknown future over the settled present, it is hard for anyone else to make very much of them, or to understand why half of them are in a foreign language. That could of course be regarded as appropriate given the general setting in which they appear. Most of Oliver Goldsmith's friends would have preferred to have had him commemorated in his own tongue but Dr Johnson, who was in charge of the matter, stoutly refused 'to disgrace the walls of Westminster Abbey with an English inscription'. All this was however in the eighteenth century. A more plausible defence of choosing from Lawrence's work a line which is only half in English is that he was himself a gifted linguist fond (sometimes over-fond) of introducing foreign phrases into his writing. In Eastwood he worked hard at his French and never afterwards seems to have had any trouble in speaking it. Living with Frieda made him fluent enough in German not only to read and talk but also to write reasonably long letters in that language to his mother-in-law. His Italian was good enough to allow him to publish several translations of Italian works and when he lived in Mexico he quickly became fluent in Spanish. But these were *modern* languages and Latin was a wholly different matter. He never read it with any ease and his knowledge became limited to a familiarity with a number of tags ('Climbing down Pisgah' is a meditation on Terence's famous *Homo sum. Humani a me alienum puto*—I am a man and therefore nothing human is alien to me). One reason for this was that Latin was not a language he could get to know better through talking but another, perhaps more important one was that it had not been beaten into him (along with Greek) at a public school. What therefore makes *homo sum* inappropriate as half of the four words celebrating Lawrence is that Latin was the *lingua franca* of the gentlemanly classes and he not only gave up very quickly any aspirations he may once have had to be an English gentleman, but was never regarded as such by others. Remembering his first meeting with him, David Garnett described Lawrence as 'slight in build, with a weak, narrow chest and shoulders . . . His hair was of a colour, and grew in a particular way, which I have never seen except in English working men. It was bright mud colour, with a streak of red in it, a thick mat, parted on one side. Somehow it was incredibly plebeian, mongrel and underbred.' These were only Garnett's *first* impressions but there must have been many who shared them and for those people it would have been yet another sign of the decline of the West that a man like Lawrence could be admitted into Westminster Abbey.

Representing a great writer with a few words from his own work is an impossible task. When opinions were being canvassed for a suitable choice in the weeks before the stone was laid, one admirer facetiously suggested 'I blame his mother' while another's more serious proposal was 'Basta, basta'. This last is also a foreign phrase but one Lawrence often used, and it is from a language which does not carry the same social connotations as Latin. It also has the advantage of suggesting both how Lawrence was worn down by his illness (one could very easily have imagined 'basta, basta' as his last words), and how he might have felt about attempts to find phrases which could sum him up. The Abbey stone could not and does not do that, but it provides an opportunity for quiet reflection on the meaning of his life and work, and an alternative location for those not in striking distance of Frieda's garish temple in New Mexico. Finding Lawrence with Lewis Carroll to his immediate right and Edward Lear now beneath him may seem incongruous, but choosing one's company is even less of an option in poet's corner than it is in the local churchyard or crematorium. For him to be just below Byron seems fitting while diagonally across from the bottom right of his own stone is the one commemorating poets from the First World War. They are named in a long list of sixteen which begins with his friend Richard Aldington and includes Robert Nichols.

The Westminster Abbey stone and Frieda's temple are both focuses for thought but a third is provided by the headstone from the graveyard in Vence. Martha Crotch hung on to this once Lawrence's body had been exhumed and in penurious old age made an unsuccessful attempt to sell it. After her death it was given to Professor de Sola Pinto of Nottingham University and has finished up behind a glass panel on the wall of the public library in Eastwood. Taos, London, and his home town are therefore all places where the Lawrence phoenix can be seen and his achievements celebrated. Enoch Soames would complain that all this attention is of little consequence to those ashes Angelo Ravagli left behind in Marseilles, just as the prospect of it would not have meant much to their owner while he was still alive. But if there is one thing that headstones, mausoleums, and memorial stones make clear it is that acts of commemoration are for the benefit of the living not the dead because it would make not the slightest sense to perform them for anyone else.

Although in his darkest days Lawrence always continued to believe that his voice would one day be heard, he was unlike Stendhal in having no very precise ideas about when that day would come, and he lived too intensely in the moment ever to concern himself unduly with how he would be regarded after his death. One of the methods writers have sometimes devised for promoting posthumous fame is to leave behind material whose subsequent publication will help keep their name alive. The appearance of *The Virgin and the Gypsy* shortly after Lawrence's death, or of a whole new novel (*Mr Noon*), more than fifty years later, could be considered in that light if he had not felt scruples about the first and if the second, occupying almost three hundred pages in the excellent Cambridge University Press edition of his complete letters and works, was writing he had never completed. The decision to lay both texts before the public, with whatever good or ill effects that might have for his reputation, was in other hands than his. In other hands also was clearly the determination of the Cambridge editors to do Lawrence posthumous justice by ridding what he wrote of all the blemishes due to censorship, human error, or misfortune at the unavoidable expense of presenting a fiercely non-academic author in texts which are heavily annotated, full of commentary, and very expensive. We cannot know what he would have felt about this, only that he had of necessity no part in the deal.

Mr Noon appeared in 1984, when the Cambridge edition was in full flow, and a year before the unveiling of the Abbey stone. This was a time when, after the boom of the 1960s and 1970s, Lawrence's reputation was beginning its decline towards its present low point and also, perhaps, when Establishment values were under such attack that an invitation to the Abbey was beginning to bring faint echoes of Groucho Marx's famous suggestion that any club willing to accept him as a member was no longer worth joining. In his welcome to those who attended the unveiling ceremony, the Dean of Westminster alluded to a series of books by Walter

Savage Landor called *Imaginary Conversations*, which he expected many of his listeners would have read. Landor is a writer who once had a vogue among the more classically educated but who has now almost completely disappeared from view. Yet any decent university library is likely to house the splendid, sixteen-volume edition of his works completed in the 1960s, one which tends to remain splendid because so few students handle it and now falls into the special enclosure posterity reserves for its white elephants. It is always possible that in the not too distant future it may be joined there by the Cambridge edition of Lawrence's works. One factor which makes this seem unlikely at present is the large number of loyal readers he still has in non-academic circles although it remains to be seen how far their British numbers will be diminished by the gradual disappearance of his books from school curricula.

'Memorialisation in Westminster Abbey', said the Dean, 'not only reflects contemporary judgement but registers a vote of confidence that succeeding generations will think likewise.' He acknowledged that the choice of his predecessors had not always proved justified but declared his own belief that the choice of D. H. Lawrence would. Yet who can anticipate the effects of such apparently trivial but in fact momentous events as changes in school curricula? Those who have thought forward to their own posthumous fame have naturally imagined it developing in circumstances much like their present ones without remembering that social or political changes take place which can have an unpredictable influence on literary reputation and on taste. If Lawrence's fame has suffered more in recent years than that of Joyce or Woolf, it is in some part because he was neither

Irish nor female. There was (that is) neither an emergent, recently independent nation's pride in its literary heritage, nor what is sometimes called the second phase of feminism, to shelter him from the belated discovery that his conceptions of a woman's role in life can often sound neanderthal and his political ideas are not exactly those of a liberal democrat. Times change and judgements change with them. 'It is doubtful', writes Raymond Tallis in an article on 'The Death of Immortality', 'whether even Shakespeare will be remembered in 40,000 AD,' and he urges us to realize that 'all our purposes converge to purposelessness and that all our mattering fades to insignificance'. Admirers of Lawrence might well protest that they are not interested in such a distant view but only (for example) in whether he will be remembered as long as there are people still interested in English literature. Yet even on that question it is perhaps as well to remember that one of the many facets of Etruscan civilization he admired was that their temples were built of wood and that therefore none of them have survived. Why has mankind such a craving to be imposed upon, he asks, in a passage which provides a suitably approximate last word on the question of his posthumous fame, 'Why this lust after imposing creeds, imposing deeds, imposing buildings, imposing language, imposing works of art? The thing becomes an imposition and a weariness at last.'

Postscript: On the Fear of Death

Only those who are extraordinary, or in extraordinary circumstances, fail to fear death. It is a fear which has at least two distinct aspects. The first and more familiar is fear of the pain of dying. This is something we all hope to minimize but know that we will be unusually fortunate to avoid altogether. One of Simone de Beauvoir's finest works is *Une mort très douce* (usually translated as *A Very Easy Death*) and describes in graphic, moving detail the death of her mother from cancer. The title of the book is taken from the words used to describe the last hours of the mother by one of the nurses who attended her. In the use de Beauvoir makes of them they are meant to be ironic and certainly this is their effect given the degree of unnecessary pain and suffering which the book records. Yet the nurse was perhaps doing no more than making a comparative judgement and saying that this patient had been able to go more gently (*doucement*) into what Dylan Thomas called the good night than many others she had seen before. Anyone with the courage to turn back again to Tolstoy's account of the death of Ivan Ilyich might agree that this could be so. In recent times it has been discovered that the body contains what have been called endorphins and that these can release tranquilizing, pain-dulling substances in moments of great stress. But a good deal of uncertainty surrounds how consistently and effectively endorphins operate and they do not seem to have done much for poor Ivan Ilyich. The only possible benefit to be found in sufferings like his is that they make death welcome.

But it is here that the second, much rarer fear becomes relevant: that of non-existence, of no longer being alive. 'I should not really object to dying', writes Thomas Nagel, 'if it were not followed by death.' Philip Larkin put it more directly when he yelled at his friend Kingsley Amis, 'I am not only frightened of dying, I'm afraid of being dead.' From a logical point of view this second fear hardly makes sense. Lucretius tried to allay it by pointing out that if the thought of not having existed before our birth was not troubling to us, then there was no need to be disturbed by the idea of not existing after death. But this argument has a false symmetry in that our non-existence before death was a condition which we happen to know from experience came to an end, and we have no such experience to rely on in the case of non-existence after death. The poet Anna Seward once had the temerity to tell Dr Johnson that it was absurd to dread non-existence, or what she called annihilation, because it was only a 'pleasing dream without a sleep'. He rightly pointed out that it was 'neither pleasing nor sleep; it is nothing', but when it was suggested by Boswell that in this case there was nothing to fear he followed up with, 'The lady confounds annihilation, which is nothing, with the apprehension of it, which is dreadful. It is in the apprehension of it that the horror of annihilation consists.' This fails to explain quite why anyone should fear non-existence or annihilation but confirms that many people in the past, some of them with unusually powerful minds, certainly have done so.

Lawrence's example is much more relevant to the first great fear than the second. He was no more fond of pain than the rest of us, once telling Catherine Carswell, 'I always thank my stars that I don't have pains that scintillate in full consciousness. I am only half there when I am ill, and so there is only half a man to suffer. To suffer in one's whole self is such a violation, that it is not to be endured.' Never robust, when he was eventually sent to school he did not join the other boys in their usual rough and tumble but preferred the company of girls, so much so that he was once followed home with his young male contemporaries chanting contemptuously, 'Dicky Dicky Denches plays with the wenches'. ('They used to say I had too much of the woman in me,' Mellors complains at one point in *Lady Chatterley's Lover*.) He missed out on the physical hardening which the traditional male sports are said to produce and one manifestation of his supposedly 'feminine' sensibility in later life was a dislike of being touched. In what was a familiar self-identification, the cry of the resurrected Jesus—*noli me tangere* or touch me not—became a favourite with him. This was after what had been the great crisis in his horror of being touched in the wrong way. Lawrence went through several medical inspections during the war but at the last of them, in Derby in 1918, it may have been that the doctors identified him as the local author of a banned book and a prominent anti-war intellectual. The way they held his testicles to check whether he had a hernia, or told him to turn round and bend over so that they could look down his anus, made him feel that they were deliberately humiliating him. When he described the experience later in his Australian novel *Kangaroo* the rage it caused was still bubbling inside him: 'Never would he be touched again.—And because they had handled his private parts, and looked into them, their eyes should burst and their hands should wither and their hearts should rot.' This reaction appears hysterical and was clearly regarded as such by the novelist J. C. Powys, who in his *Autobiography* writes: 'In the recruiting room I was looked over just in the way D. H. Lawrence in *Kangaroo* so indignantly describes himself as being, but as I have almost as deep a "feminine" penchant for doctors as I have for priests I did not mind at all!' His surprising comment not only invites us to reconsider what might in fact have been a 'normal' reaction to the indignities Lawrence felt he had suffered but also suggests how imprecise or misleading a description of his temperament as feminine might be. What the Derby experience does help to make clearer, however, is why he should later have been always so reluctant to put himself in the power of doctors he did not know.

Lawrence's behaviour during his boyhood and youth led to his sometimes being called a 'mardarse' ('mard' being a dialect word for soft), but no one who crossed him in those days would have thought the term accurate. Highly strung can also often mean highly irritable and the explosions of rage to which he was prone would make him entirely indifferent to his own physical security. Too unathleetic and lightly built to chastise others with his fists, he had a power of invective which would often leave his antagonists dazed and feeling that they would have preferred the weight of a hand much heavier than his than to have to listen to his abuse. These outbursts continued into adulthood so that it is surprising that there is only one recorded instance of his being hit (other of course than by Frieda). When they were provoked by genuine grievances or injustices, which was by no means always the case, they represented examples of the kind of moral courage which cannot function effectively without a good deal of the physical variety also. This might suggest that Lawrence could only demonstrate that he was not in fact a mardarse when he abandoned self-control, but the opposite was true in his dealings with his illness. Frieda's main emphasis after his death was on the dignity with which her husband died and she expressed gratitude that he had remained in control until the very end (of Katherine Mansfield she said that she 'was so disciplined in so many things, but I think she let herself go in her being ill'). 'He faced the end so splendidly, so like a *man*', Frieda told an American friend ten days after Lawrence had died. Her tone always tended to suggest that he had stoically endured those sufferings which he had described to Catherine Carswell as unendurable largely for her benefit; but there may have been some truth in that. She was a professional soldier's daughter, brought up among soldiers in the garrison town of Metz, and had a high regard for manliness, describing Lawrence's face in death as 'so proud, manly and splendid'. His efforts to make himself less of the woman some of his contemporaries in Eastwood had thought him, and more of the kind of man Frieda had been conditioned to admire, may well have influenced the way he faced up to death and all the pain it entailed.

The relevance of Lawrence to the second way of fearing death is minimal because he hardly ever seems to have experienced it. This was probably not because he was fully and imaginatively possessed of the absurdity of apprehending a condition in which nothing can ever harm or trouble us again. When in *Measure for Measure* the young Claudio is having second thoughts about sacrificing his life for his sister and says, 'Ay, but to die, and go we know not where, | To lie in cold obstruction, and to rot', he is speaking in terms everyone accepts and understands. Yet of course once he was dead he would not know that the obstruction in which he lay was cold or how many worms were making their way through his rotting corpse. The mistake is similar to the one Anna Seward makes when she talks of annihilation being like sleep and it consists of confusing non-being with any recognizable human state involving a temporary rather than permanent absence of consciousness. The 'oblivion' Lawrence sometimes yearns for appears to have been just such a state. In the early 1920s he wrote a satirical short story called 'Smile' in which he described a figure very like Middleton Murry going to see a woman very like Katherine Mansfield, a woman who (in the version he always favoured of the real events on which the story is modelled) was already dead. To avoid too obvious an identification, the man is travelling not to Fontainebleau but to a convent in Rome where his wife has died. As he does so he cannot help repeating to himself the second stanza of a poem by Thomas Hood called 'The Death-Bed'. This had appeared in the late nineteenth century's favourite anthology, Palgrave's *Golden Treasury*, a copy of which (Jessie Chambers reports) was always in Lawrence's pocket when he was in his late teens. In its correct version (working from memory Lawrence slightly misquotes) the stanza goes:

> But when the morn came dim and sad
> And chill with early showers,
> Her quiet eyelids closed—she had
> Another morn than ours.

The hero of 'Smile' is described as having a 'critical mind' and he therefore feels contempt for what he calls the bathos of this poem's ending, and 'even self-contempt' for having remembered it. Yet, however contemptible Hood's rhythm and diction may be, it is only from a literary point of view that his ending is an anticlimax. If there were indeed 'another morn' then no one's life could end in bathos, whatever else its conclusion might be. As 'The Ship of Death' suggests, Lawrence's oblivion usually carries with it at least a hint of another morn.

Lawrence seems to have been someone who lived so intensely from day to day that he could not conceive the future as a blank. The fear of non-being which derives from imagining what it might be to have, as Larkin puts in 'Aubade', 'no sight, no sound, | No touch or taste or smell, nothing to think with' was largely foreign to him. For most of his life he was driven on by a sense of mission. When in New Mexico he was being asked by the journalist why he wrote, part of his answer was that it 'would be wrong, entirely wrong, to possess a talent and have thoughts without sharing them with the world'. His use of a word which would remind most readers of the resulting interview of what Jesus had to say about talents in the parable of that name was probably no accident. But like other writers who have felt they have many thoughts to share, he was sometimes conscious of living on borrowed time. Catherine Carswell was five years older than Lawrence but he once casually told her that of course she had many more years before her than he had. There was a paradoxical sense in which he did not expect to live long, but always a little longer. In that way he would avoid not only oblivion but also the possibility of what Larkin calls, again in 'Aubade', the 'total emptiness for ever, | The sure extinction that we travel to | And shall be lost in always.'

How Lawrence was remembered has an obvious relevance for anyone concerned with the nature of grief or the problem of funerals and memorials, but the interest of the way he faced the fear of death, in either of its major forms, might seem compromised by his being such an unusual human being. His genetic make-up, and the circumstances of his upbringing, made him exceptional in so many ways that it could seem futile to attempt to draw lessons from his example. Those who wrote the lives of the saints were able to draw such lessons because most of what they said about their subjects was invented, but modern biographers are committed to being as historically accurate as possible. The more minutely circumstantial they manage to be, the more individual their subjects are likely to appear and the less their behaviour can be made to fall into usefully exemplary patterns. In 1912, during the euphoria of having completed what he believed to be the final version of *Sons and Lovers*, Lawrence wrote, 'it's the tragedy of thousands of young men in England'. A modern reader might be inclined to wonder whether the hero of this novel is quite that representative and yet, in the same year, Freud published a paper in which he described how certain young men who are devoted to their mothers develop such an elevated notion of womanhood that they find it impossible to have proper sexual feelings for any of the respectable young girls of their own generation, that there is therefore in them a fatal split between physical and spiritual love. The title he gave to this essay has been translated as 'The most prevalent form of degradation in erotic life'. The prevalence of the degradation in question, or of the kind of difficulties Paul Morel experiences, may of course have been no more than period phenomena which have been swept away in the climate of sexual permissiveness Lawrence's own *Lady Chatterley's Lover* inadvertently did so much to promote. Yet on this question of what remains representative and therefore instructive for us all, it is important not to work with the wrong model. We tend to think of ourselves as stable creatures to whom the experience of reading a novel or a biography can simply be bolted on, according to its greater or lesser degree of relevance. Yet it might often be truer to say that we are a cluster of potentialities and that knowledge of someone else's experience, whether it is conveyed through fiction or biographical writing, can therefore more easily inform and lead into new places what Lawrence calls in *Lady Chatterley's Lover* 'the flow of our sympathetic consciousness'. In any case, just as there are no legs so short that they don't reach the ground, so there are no human beings so individual that they are not at the same time representative in many respects.

The experience of even such an unusual human being as D. H. Lawrence can matter in that, although fear of death may take diverse forms, everyone's life is determined by the anxious knowledge, more or less recognized or suppressed, that death will one day come. Attempting to justify his claim that there 'has rarely passed a life of which a judicious and faithful narrative would not be useful', Dr Johnson said that 'we are all prompted by the same motives, all deceived by the same fallacies, all animated by hope, obstructed by danger, entangled by desire, and seduced by pleasure'. This makes human experience sound far more uniform than we now believe it to be, but Johnson would have been wholly justified in adding to his list that we all know, or should know, that we will one day die. As the psalmist says, 'What man is he that liveth, and shall not see death?'

Acknowledgements and Sources

I am very grateful to my collaborators on the Cambridge biography of Lawrence, John Worthen and Mark Kinkead-Weekes, for long years of friendship and support. John Worthen kindly read a first draft of this book, correcting several errors and making many valuable suggestions. For other suggestions, especially of a philosophical variety, I am heavily indebted to Frank Cioffi. Eldon Pethybridge and Brenda Sumner provided me with valuable legal information and Andrew Johnson, a consultant at the Kent and Canterbury hospital, generously took time off from a busy life to put me right on several matters concerning tuberculosis. The expert on Lawrence's time in Vence, and on the later exhumation of his body, is Émile Delavenay. I am very grateful to his widow Katherine for much useful information and for the loan of some of her husband's papers. Angela Faunch and her colleagues in the Document Delivery department of the Templeman Library of Kent University have as usual been most cooperative; and I have received active support from Dorothy Johnston, who is the keeper of the manuscripts and special collections in the university library at Nottingham. For various other kinds of help I would like to thank Sheila Bell, Edward Greenwood, Michael Holroyd, Hermione Lee, Deborah Matthews, Christopher Pollnitz, Peter Preston, Hugh Ridley,

Claire Tomalin, Jenny Uglow, John Wiltshire, and my wife Geneviève. All errors of scholarship or of taste are my own.

The sources for any biographical study of Lawrence begin with his letters, in either Aldous Huxley's 1932 edition, the collection in two volumes edited by Harry T. Moore in 1962, or the splendid eight volumes of the Cambridge edition whose general editor is James T. Boulton (Cambridge, 1979–2000). The three volumes of Edward Nehls's *Composite Biography* of Lawrence (Madison, Wisc., 1957–9) are invaluable and, as far as more orthodox life-writing is concerned, I have naturally relied a good deal on the Cambridge biography: John Worthen's *Early Years* (1991), Mark Kinkead-Weekes's *Triumph to Exile* (1996), and my own *Dying Game* (1998). There are very useful biographies of Frieda by Robert Lucas (London, 1973) and Janet Byrne (London, 1995), and much additional information in *Living at the Edge: A Biography of D. H. Lawrence and Frieda von Richthofen* by Michael Squires and Lynn K. Talbot (London, 2002). Many of her letters were published in *Frieda Lawrence: The Memoirs and Correspondence* edited by E. W. Tedlock (London, 1961) and in Harry T. Moore and Dale B. Montague's *Frieda Lawrence and her Circle* (London, 1981); but John Worthen and Cornelia Rumpf-Worthen have shown me their translations of Frieda's letters to her mother, Lawrence's surviving niece, Joan King, kindly allowed me to see letters written by Frieda to Lawrence's sister Emily, and there is important information about her in three letters from Mabel Luhan to her friend Una Jeffers, which are in the Bancroft Library of the University of California in Berkeley. These are the general sources for material in this book; more specific attributions are given in the following notes, where the place of publication is London unless otherwise stated.

INTRODUCTION AND PART I

(p. x) 'the religious journals': see the account of exemplary deaths in *Death in the Victorian Family* (Oxford, 1996) by Pat Jalland, who acknowledges, as do all those who have tried to think about attitudes to death, the pioneer work of the French scholar Philippe Ariès; (p. xii) 'some philosophers': there is excellent material in the anthology on *Immortality* edited by Paul Edwards in 1997 and published in Amherst, New York; Freud's remark occurs in 'Thoughts for the Times on War and Death', first published in 1915; (p. xiv) Carey's review appeared in the *Sunday Times* on 24 April 1983 and Larkin's in the *Observer* on the same date; (p. 3) 'like a bad smell': the quotations are from two late poems by Lawrence, 'The Greeks are coming!' and 'The Argonauts'; (p. 6) 'their old friend, Norman Douglas': unless otherwise indicated remarks on Lawrence by his friends or relatives can usually be found in Nehls's *Composite Biography*; Lawrence is sarcastic about central heating in his essay 'Pan in America'; (p. 8) 'Knud Merrild': see his *A Poet and Two Painters* (1938); (p. 10) 'registered deaths from tuberculosis': there is a long list of excellent books on tuberculosis—my chief sources have been R. Y. Keers, *Pulmonary Tuberculosis: A Journey down the Centuries* (1978), Linda Bryder, *Below the Magic Mountain: A Social History of Tuberculosis in Twentieth-Century Britain* (Oxford, 1980), and Frank Ryan, *Tuberculosis: The Greatest Story Never Told* (Bromsgrove, 1992);

(p. 12) for details here see *Mark Gertler* by Sarah Macdougall (2002) and *Willie: The Life of Somerset Maugham* by Robert Calder (1989); 'a less fortunate and closer friend': the best biography among several very good ones of Katherine Mansfield is by Claire Tomalin, published in 1987; (p. 16) 'David Garnett': see his memoir *The Golden Echo*, first published in 1954; (p. 17) 'a text book of the time': Andrew Morland, *Pulmonary Tuberculosis in General Practice* (1932); (pp. 18–19) for details here see Bernard Crick, *George Orwell* (1980) and Leslie A. Marchand, *Byron: A Portrait* (1971); (p. 20) Sorescu's poem can be found in *The Oxford Book of Death*; (p. 29) 'the letter from early 1920': this letter no longer exists but reports from Middleton Murry of its contents are reliable. There is a thorough investigation of its context in Mark Kinkead-Weekes's *Triumph to Exile*; (p. 30) 'one medical authority's': i.e. Dr N. D. C. Lewis, cited by Leslie A. Marchand in *Byron: A Biography* (1957); (p. 36) 'not anything that should be felt of': the strange English does not indicate anything peculiar about Herr Ferge's German but is a characteristic idiosyncrasy of H. T. Lowe-Porter, Mann's translator; (p. 42) Chekhov and TB: see the biography by Donald Rayfield (New York, 1997); (p. 43) most of my information about Wells comes from the admirable biography by Norman and Jeanne Mackenzie (1973); (p. 45) 'Major C. H. Stevens': see E. Ernst, 'Stevens' Cure: A Secret Remedy', *Journal of the Royal Society of Medicine* (September 2002); (p. 48) for details of Else see Martin Green, *The Von Richthofen Sisters* (1974); (p. 50) Kafka's 'obscure welcome' is a suggestion in Ronald Hayman's 1981 biography of him; (p. 55) 'Catherine Carswell describes': in *The Savage Pilgrimage: A Narrative of D. H. Lawrence* (1932); (p. 57)

Nietzsche's remarks on Schopenhauer are in *The Genealogy of Morals*; 'Huxley's view': in the introduction to the 1932 edition of Lawrence's letters; (p. 58) 'National Association for the Prevention of Tuberculosis': cited in Linda Bryder's *Below the Magic Mountain*; (pp. 60–1) Maugham's story was called 'Sanatorium' and first published in 1938; (p. 64) 'as Pascal approached death': see Michel Schneider, *Morts imaginaires* (Paris, 2003); the Archbishop's comments can be found in the *Daily Telegraph* Saturday Review, 20 August 2005; (p. 65) 'Theosophy': there is an excellent account of this movement in Peter Washington's *Madame Blavatsky's Baboon* (New York, 1993); there are detailed description of Yeats's involvement in Theosophy in the biographies by Richard Ellmann (1949) and Roy Foster (Oxford, 1997, 2003); Blake's remark occurs in *Jerusalem* (1804); (p. 68) Lawrence's 'Almond Blossom' appears in his collection *Birds, Beasts and Flowers*; (p. 69) 'Immortality Ode': properly of course 'Intimations of Immortality from Recollections of Early Childhood'. Wordsworth's note reads: 'I was often unable to think of material things as having external existence ... Many times while going to school have I grasped at a wall or tree to recall myself from this abyss of idealism'; (p. 70) 'Schopenhauer once commented': in his *The World as Will and Idea* (1818); (p. 75) in addition to Robert Gitting's biography of Keats (1970) I have consulted the more recent work by Stephen Coote (1995); (p. 77) 'religious scruples': there is an account of these in *The Savage God: A Study of Suicide* by A. Alvarez (1971); (p. 78) 'Spencer': in *The Fairy Queen*, bk. 1, canto 9, stanza 40; (p. 80) 'Dorothy Parker': see her poem 'Résumé' in *Not so deep as a well* (1937).

PART II

(p. 89) 'Compton Mackenzie...acquired two of them': in 1920 Mackenzie had secured the lease of Herm and Jethou in the Channel Islands; (p. 90) 'Mark Gertler had been urged by Koteliansky': see the selected letters of Gertler, edited by Noel Carrington (1965) and Koteliansky's papers which are in the British Library and include letters from Gertler, Andrew Morland, Jessie Chambers, and Lawrence's sister Ada, as well as from Lawrence himself; (p. 91) Dorothy Morland left an unpublished account of her visit which is now in the Nottinghamshire Archives; (p. 93) 'the wife of Robert Louis Stevenson': see *RLS: A Life Study* by Jenni Calder (1980); (p. 94) for details of Montaigne's death, and that of many other French writers, I have been reliant on Michel Schneider's excellent *Morts imaginaires*; (p. 98) Freud's remark about the kettle (a little more complicated than I make it seem) occurs in *The Interpretation of Dreams*; (p. 101) 'a letter from Madinier': in the Nottinghamshire Archives; (p. 102) 'Morland was wondering': one of Morland's letters to Gertler and three to Koteliansky were published by George J. Zytaruk in the first number of the *D. H. Lawrence Review* (1968); (p. 111) 'a Lawrence whom Huxley described': a generous collection of Huxley's letters was edited by Grover Smith in 1969 while the best biography of him is still probably Sybille Bedford's (1974); (p. 112) 'Maugham from later describing': in his *Introduction to Modern English and American Literature* (Garden City, New York, 1943); (p. 118) the details about Flaubert and Maupassant are from Schneider's *Morts imaginaires*; (p. 123) 'demonstrably not his': the doodles are written on a compliments slip from the *New English Weekly* which did not begin publication until 1932—see my own 'Lawrence and the Death-Bed Doodles', *Journal of D. H. Lawrence Studies*, 2 (2008); (p. 124) for Henry James see Leon Edel's biography (New York, 1978); the reference to Pushkin is in Schneider, *Morts imaginaires*; (p. 126) 'the records of Chekhov's death': these are often conflicting—see Janet Malcolm's *Reading Chekhov: A Critical Journey* (2001) and the final chapter in Hermione Lee's *Body Parts: Essays in Life-Writing* (2005); (p. 132) 'one biographer': Neville Williams in *Elizabeth: Queen of England* (1967); (p. 133) Tichbourne's poem can be found in the *New Oxford Book of English Verse*, edited by Helen Gardner (Oxford, 1972); (p. 140) Karl Marx's remark is in most anthologies of famous last words (many of which need to be shelved under fiction); (p. 141) 'Hugh Kingsmill': Hesketh Pearson reported to Michael Holroyd that Kingsmill made this remark about commas and semicolons during his final period in hospital; (p. 144) there are useful details about Nichols in *Putting Poetry First: A Life of Robert Nichols* by Anne and William Charlton (Norwich, 2003); (p. 147) for several details of Budgen and his letter describing the funeral I am reliant on an article by Christopher Pollnitz in the *Journal of the D. H. Lawrence Society* for 1997 (' "No Form or Appropriate Ceremony": An Account of D. H. Lawrence's Funeral'); (p. 150) 'disordered mourning': the phrase is often associated with John Bowlby; 'one of his early poems': 'Hymn to Priapus'; (p. 151) 'our social comforts drop away': Johnson's poem is entitled 'On the Death of Dr Robert Levet'; (p. 156) 'I can read him like a book': the passage occurs in remarks on Hawthorne's *Scarlet Letter* in Lawrence's *Studies in Classic American Literature*; (p. 157) 'only recorded statement of frank apology,: see the letter written to Louie on 19 November 1912; (p. 158) John Worthen describes his discovery of Louie's correspondence with Wells in 'Orts and Slarts: Two Biographical Pieces on D. H. Lawrence', *RES* NS, 46/181 (1995); (p. 163) the death of the narrator's grandmother occurs in the *Côté de Guermantes* section of Proust's novel.

PART III AND POSTSCRIPT

(p. 167) 'Shakespeare himself made a will': the best account is in Samuel Schoenbaum's *Shakespeare's Lives* (Oxford, 1991); (p. 171) 'Una Jeffers': wife of the poet Robinson Jeffers who, after Lawrence had left Taos, replaced him as Mabel's literary guru; (p. 172) George Lawrence's reminiscences were recorded by David Gerard in the 1960s (as were those of his son, Ernest); the tapes are in the Nottingham public library; (p. 178) the still standard biography of Murry is by F. A. Lea (1959); (p. 181) information about Frieda's 'friend Martha Crotch' comes chiefly from two slim books published by the Tragara Press in Edinburgh, her own *Memories of Frieda Lawrence* (1975) and *Some Letters of Pino Orioli to Mrs Gordon Crotch* (1974). The latter has a useful introduction by Mark Holloway, the excellent biographer of Norman Douglas; (p. 183) 'reinforced her position as a disinterested broker': this offer of Ada's is in a letter she wrote to Koteliansky, now in the British Library. Other letters of hers were published in Moore and Montague's *Frieda Lawrence and her Circle* (1981); 'what her lawyers did': it is impossible to be clear about all the details of the dispute because Frieda's correspondence with her solicitor C. H. Medley, which she refers to in a letter written to Murry in the early 1950s and which was described by Tedlock as being among her papers when she died, has gone missing; 'the hearing which was eventually held in early November': see the report in *The Times* for 4 November 1932; (p. 186) 'Dr Johnson writes interestingly': the phrases are from a letter to Mrs Thrale written in April 1776; (p. 188) 'Frieda negotiated the sale of a manuscript': see *D. H. Lawrence's Manuscripts: The Correspondence of Frieda Lawrence, Jake Zeitlin and Others*, edited by Michael Squires (1991); (p. 190) 'the second Earl of Southampton': the details can be found in *Shakespeare and the Earl of Southampton* by G. P. V. Akrigg (1968); (p. 191) 'Burns, for example': the particulars of his and other literary estates are very interestingly described in Ian Hamilton's *Keepers of the Flame: Literary Estates and the Rise of Biography* (1992); Stendhal's *testaments* are grouped together at the end of the second volume of his *Oeuvres intimes* (Paris, 1982), edited by V. Del Litto, and details of his life can be found in Michel Crouzet's *Stendhal ou Monsieur Moi-Même* (Paris, 1990); (p. 194) many of the obituaries of Lawrence are collected in *D. H. Lawrence: The Critical Heritage*, edited by R. P. Draper (1970); (p. 199) Jonathan Miller tells the story of his son's remark in *The Ruffian on the Stair: Reflections on Death*, edited by Rosmary Dinnage (1990); (p. 200) Wordsworth's remarks occur in his *Essays upon Epitaphs* (1810); (p. 201) the two volumes of Osborne's autobiography, *A Better Class of Person* and *Almost a Gentleman*, were published together in 1999 as *Looking Back: Never Explain, Never Apologise*; (p. 205) Murry's *Jesus, Man of Genius* had appeared in 1926; (p. 206) 'an account which Jessie Chambers had already written': there is an invaluable collection of 'Letters and Documents of Jessie Chambers Wood' (Wood being her married name) in the second volume of Émile Delavenay's *D. H. Lawrence: L'Homme et la genèse de son oeuvre* (Paris, 1969); (p. 221) information on the German cultural background comes from Martin Green's book—see the note to p. 48 above (p. 223) 'screwed anything he could': the view of the bibliographer Larry Powell as reported by Michael Squires in *D. H. Lawrence's Manuscripts*; (p. 226) as Doris Langley Moore demonstrates so well in *The Late Lord Byron* (1977) Trelawny is a very untrustworthy biographer but the main lines of his account of the cremation seem to be accurate; (p. 229) 'Madame de Sevigné': the detail is in Schneider's *Morts imaginaires* 'those who met de Haulleville': these include Katherine and Émile Delavenay and the whole matter is expertly reviewed in the latter's 'A Shrine without Relics', *D. H. Lawrence Review*, 18 (1983); (p. 230) for Elisabeth Nietzsche see H. F. Peters, *Zarathustra's Sister* (New York, 1977); (p. 235) 'Addison's witty remark': quoted in G. E. Troutbeck, *Westminster Abbey* (1900); (p. 239) 'Dr Johnson . . . in charge of the matter': the dispute over the inscription for Goldsmith belongs to the summer of 1776; the version of Terence's claim which Lawrence quotes in his essay reads: 'Homo sum. Omnis a me humanum alienum puto'; (p. 244) Raymond Tallis's essay appeared in *PN Review*, 170 (2006); (p. 245) 'endorphins': see Sherwin B. Noland's often harrowing *How We Die: Reflections on Life's Final Chapter* (1993); (p. 246) Thomas Nagel's phrase is quoted in *Death's Door: Modern Dying and the Ways We Grieve* by Sandra M. Gilbert (New York, 2006); 'yelled at his friend Kingsley Amis': the episode is described in Amis's *Memoirs* (1991); Anna Seward's exchanges with Johnson took place in 1778 and are recorded in Boswell; (p. 248) 'one recorded episode of his being hit': the episode is dramatized in the chapter of *Aaron's Rod* called 'A Punch in the Wind' and its source in real life is discussed by John Turner in vol. 28 of the *D. H. Lawrence Review* (1999); (p. 253) 'Dr Johnson said': *Rambler 60*, 13 October 1750 'Dignity and Uses of Biography'.

Index